The Sharp End Of The Needle
(Dealing With Diabetes, Dialysis, Transplant And The Medical Field)

Gabriel of Urantia

The Sharp End Of The Needle
(Dealing With Diabetes, Dialysis, Transplant And The Medical Field)

Gabriel of Urantia

Including selected articles from
the *Alternative Voice* periodical

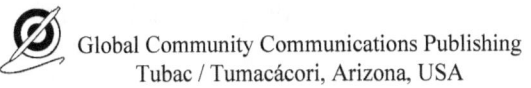
Global Community Communications Publishing
Tubac / Tumacácori, Arizona, USA

© 2012 Global Community Communications Alliance
21 20 19 18 17 16 15 14   2 3 4 5

All rights reserved. No part of this book shall be reproduced, translated, or transmitted in any form or by any means, electronic, mechanical, magnetic, photographic including photocopying, recording, or by any information storage and retrieval system, without prior written permission of Global Community Communications Publishing. No patent liability is assumed with respect to the use of the information contained herein. Although every precaution has been taken in the preparation of this book, the publisher and author assume no responsibility for errors or omissions. Neither is any liability assumed for damages resulting from the use of the information contained herein.

ISBN 978-1-937919-07-8

Global Community Communications Publishing
P.O. Box 1613, Tubac, Arizona 85646 USA
(520) 603-9932
e-mail: info@gccpublishing.org
gccpublishing.org

My gratitude to Ionia Redman
for all her work in book layout & design. Ionia has a
Bachelor of Science from Michigan State University.

My appreciation to LaTaYea Calviero,
my private secretary, typist, and grammar coach, who has a
Bachelor of Arts from Pennsylvania State University.

ABOUT THE PAPER USED IN THIS BOOK

According to our printer, Lightning Source, Inc. has 'Chain of Custody' certifications with The Sustainable Forestry Initiative, The Forest Stewardship Council, and The Programme for the Endorsement of Forest Certification that permit Lightning Source to complete the custody chain from the stump, to the mill, to the paper, to the finished books. No papers used in Lightning Source books are sourced from endangered old growth forests, forests of exceptional conservation value, or the Amazon Basin.

*I wrote this book
so people would not
have to go through
the pain and suffering
I went through.*

*The book is
a teaching tool
for preventative health.*

— Gabriel of Urantia

CONTENTS

In Gratitude x

Introduction xii

Preface xiii

Foreword: The Medical Field xv

Dedication xviii

PART 1 — The Sharp End Of The Needle (Dealing With Diabetes, Dialysis, Transplant And The Medical Field)
A Series of Journals 1

Song Lyrics: *The Sharp End Of The Needle* 59

Experiencing The Aftermath Of The January 8, 2011 Shooting Of Gabrielle Giffords 60

Journals Continued 66

DeleVan's Experience As The Donor 70

Appeal For More Organ Transplant Research And Artificial Organ Transplants 76

Final Journals 79

PART 2 — The High Cost Of Healthcare:
From Babies To Hospice, From the *Alternative Voice*, a quarterly periodical designed to sharpen the minds of higher thinkers 109

Eco-Systems, Social-Systems, And Person-Systems
by Niánn Emerson Chase 112

The Truth and Answers About Free Healthcare
by Gabriel of Urantia 120

The Medical Industrial Complex
by Marayeh Cunningham, Ph.D., Clinical Psychologist 130

My Fellow Doctors And Patients The World Over, Mortal Strugglers All, Let Us Unite In The Universal Health-Giver of All—God—For Goodness' Sake
by Landau Lawrence, M.D. 149

Hospice—A Winning Situation
by Aládi Goodman, R.N., CHPN 157

The Gesundheit! Hospital Project
by Patch Adams, M.D. 163

Pills
by Minister LaTaYea Calviero 180

Soulistic Medical Institute — A Nonprofit Organization
by Marayeh Cunningham, Ph.D.,
Clinical Psychologist 186

Book Review of *Teachings On Healing, From A Spiritual Perspective*
by Minister Lah-May Bremer,
Hospice I.T. Administrator 196

Reference Notes 198

About the Author 202

Gabriel of Urantia's
Service Ministry Experience 204

Global Community Communications Alliance   209

Seminars, Workshops & Internships 218

Alliance Organizations 220

All proceeds from
the sale of this book go to the
Personality Integration Rehabilitation
Program for Teens and Adults,
founded by Gabriel of Urantia and
Niánn Emerson Chase
(pirp.info)
and Avalon Gardens
agricultural internships
(avalongardens.org)

IN GRATITUDE

I want to especially thank these three men. Their combined effort, experience, and knowledge definitely got me off dialysis and most likely saved my life.

The University of Arizona Medical Center

Rainer W.G. Gruessner, M.D., FACS
Chairman, Department of Surgery
Chief, Division of Abdominal Transplant
Director, HepatoPancreaticoBiliary Center
Professor of Surgery and Immunology

Bruce Kaplan, M.D.
Medical Director, Transplant Nephrology

Kasturi Vinay Ranga, M.D.
Transplant Nephrology

In gratitude to **Jeanette Dinning**, RN and Transplant Case Manager, who was very helpful in explaining what we needed to do in regards to my insurance coverage. She was always available either by phone or email, which helped expedite the transplant process literally from dialysis to kidney transplant in a timing and professional manner. She is also in an important position to follow the post-transplant patient for a year straight, as she did with personal caring direct phone calls, answering questions, and giving helpful directions and suggestions along the way.

I'm additionally grateful to **Annette Whinery**, Transplant Coordinator, who was right there always for myself and my wife in trying to move the transplant forward as professionally as possible, through the red tape and human errors, which could have slowed down the transplant-acquirement process. She was a beautiful example of what a career nurse should be—personable, genuinely caring, and always returning your phone calls, knowing that you are in a tender place in time.

I also want to thank **Dr. Joy L. Logan**, nephrologist at Arizona Kidney Disease & Hypertension Center, who I see regularly and who checks my blood tests each month and gives other good advice on how to keep my 22-year-old kidney.

I want to thank **April Nelson** formerly of Davita Dialysis Center in Nogales, Arizona, and all the wonderful staff (who sometimes sing in Spanish as they work), and all the wonderful Mexican people I met there. They were real people. She is now working at DaVita Pascua Yaqui Tribe in Tucson, Arizona.

I also want to thank **Lynette Jahner, R.N., BSN**, of Fresenius Medical Care in Tucson, Arizona, who takes personal interest in her patients, is very experienced, and I always felt good with her, even taking blood from my arm. She was very loving and has a faith in God. She is now at the Grant Road facility of Fresenius Medical Care in Tucson.

INTRODUCTION

While I was on dialysis, I told the head nurse, of more than twenty-five years' experience, that I was writing a book on my dialysis experience, called *The Sharp End Of The Needle*. She told me there is also a Web site and several articles by that name that I might want to research, and so I did. All of the articles have good information and are worth reading. The site is by Bill Peckham and is called Dialysis From The Sharp End Of The Needle (bill-peckham.com). Bill Peckham is also a dialysis patient who has had a transplant, lost the kidney, and is presently on home dialysis.

Where I grew up in Pittsburgh, Pennsylvania, the term "sharp end of the needle" was used among drug addicts and being in rehabilitation ministry for many years, this term was very familiar to me. When I got on dialysis, I realized why this term is used among dialysis patients. If you type "The Sharp End Of The Needle" in on the Internet, other articles will come up.

PREFACE

I wrote this book like a journal, expressing what I felt at the time: the shock of losing my kidneys and the fear of going on dialysis with my survival relying on machines that transferred my blood out of my body through them and then back into my body—3 days a week, 4 hours per day. I wrote about my immediate experiences in the hospitals and the different dialysis centers. I wrote about the good doctors, nurses, and social service workers I experienced and the bad and uncaring ones. I tried to pull no punches because I felt I wanted other dialysis patients who read this, as well as people with any disease, to be aware of the kinds of situations they will have to face under the present health care system and how to not only deal with the health care system and practitioners but to have hope and faith in God to get them through it. That is how I got through it.

114,000 people are awaiting organ donations.
18 people die each day.
100 million are registered donors
but millions more are needed
because the donor has to be the right match.

— organdonor.gov

FOREWORD: THE MEDICAL FIELD

In the medical field, everything is connected to making money. It hasn't always been that way. Most doctors really used to be concerned about healing people. Now there are just a few of the tens of thousands of doctors who are really concerned about the patient and just not their pocketbooks. The cost of paying loans back for young practitioners just out of medical school is a chain that locks them into the greedy system that often takes half a lifetime to pay off, if ever. The medical system is set up that physicians have to go back to school every so often and pay to learn something they'll probably never use. It's the same with massage therapists and other healing practitioners.

Psychiatrists are the worst culprits of being disconnected to really being able to heal anyone today. They are connected to the A.M.A. (the American Medical Association) and the pharmaceutical companies. It's a several-hundred-billion-dollar connection to the pharmaceutical companies. The psychiatrists have developed hundreds of new disorders that they diagnose for patients, for which there is a new pill to prescribe. Medicare and Medicaid often have to pay for it, and the government allows it because certain politicians and lawmakers also benefit financially from subsidies and kickbacks from corporations of the medical industrial complex.

These psychotropic meds can create mindless drugged zombies who won't be able to really get an education to think for themselves because the fallen system needs slaves to work menial and manual labor jobs. Stalin and Hitler murdered millions of people. America drugs them and keeps them medicated with "legal" drugs.

Today, psychiatry often diagnoses free-thinking individuals (who think outside of the mainstream mindset) as "bipolar" or by some other personality-disorder label. Free-thinkers united in some form of group are often called "cults." Throughout history these free-thinkers have been burned at the stake by those in the power-elite who feared their free thinking, afraid that they will oppose the power-elite's insidious plans to make money off of the "common folk." Today doctors are addicting school children by prescribing legal drugs, which cause more psychological problems than heal them.

I, of course, realize that some medications and drugs are necessary to heal the body's many systems, but in the field of psychiatry I have my doubts if any drug is actually necessary to heal the mind and soul. The Soulistic Medical Institute—which I co-founded along with Niánn Emerson Chase (a descendant of Ralph Waldo Emerson, who was a minister, an alternative thinker, and definitely connected to the Source of light)—uses a method in counseling called "morontia counseling," which addresses the soul/mind without the need to prescribe any drug or diagnose someone with a mental illness.

I strongly suggest that you view the documentary film *Making a Killing: The Untold Story of Psychotropic Drugging*, which has to do with how psychiatry and the pharmaceutical companies are keeping teenagers and young adults, by the tens of thousands, addicted to drugs in both civilian life and the military. To learn more about the film, contact the Citizens Commission on Human Rights (cchr.org).

In this book you will see that I have mixed feelings, because I met—all through my illness—people who belonged in the medical field and people who did not. Often sometimes you just have to grin and bear it and pray to the Creator that there will be a better world to come.

DEDICATION

I dedicate this book to two precious souls, who you might say kept me alive: my wife TiyiEndea and my daughter DeleVan.

TiyiEndea — She was with me when the doctor told me I had two kidneys that were both acute and chronic—in other words, gone beyond repair. We went right to the Emergency Room together, and she was like my female Lancelot and Florence Nightingale, all rolled into one. TiyiEndea took care of everything—doctors, nurses, cleaning me, feeding me, attending to it all. And for the next eight months she drove me to dialysis three times a week, sat by my side while there, and held my hand when the nurses were trying to find my veins with these huge 1" needles. She was my caretaker in post-surgery after my kidney transplant and had to remember all the immunosuppressant drugs that I was taking. She still continues to attend to my needs and handles all contacts with all the doctors I see. I will have to take these immunosuppressant drugs for the rest of my life unless I can someday get an artificial kidney (which scientists are working on).

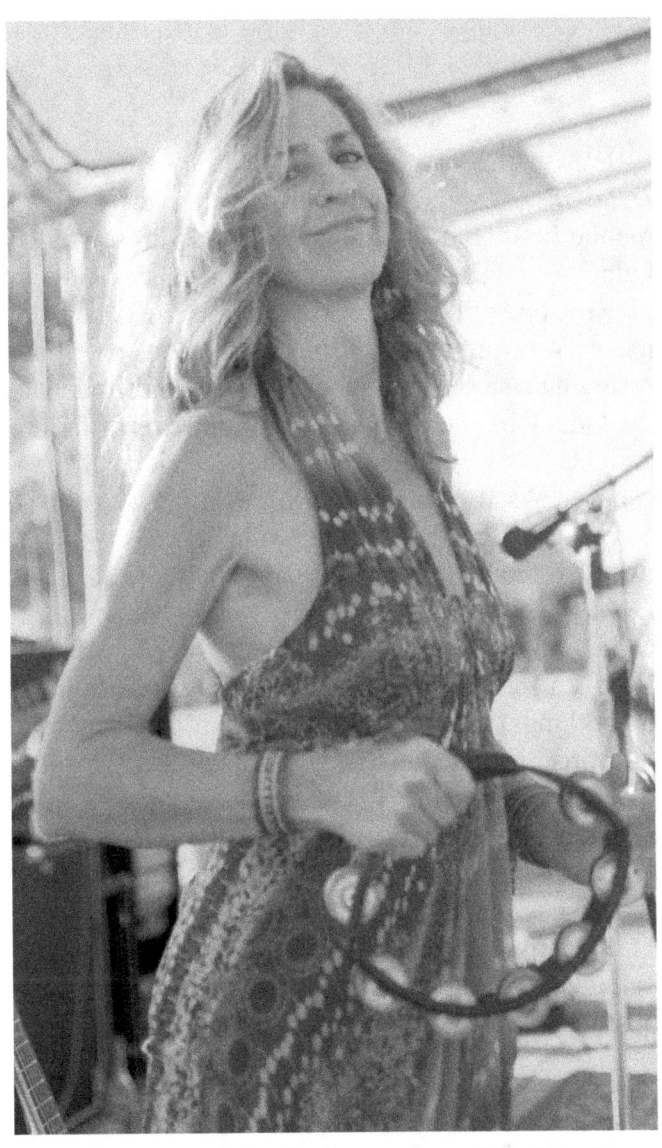

My wife and main caregiver, TiyiEndea

DeleVan — My 22-year-old daughter who visited me the first day I was in the hospital with my failed kidneys and immediately told me that she wanted to give me one of her kidneys. This gave me hope from the very beginning. I did not have to worry about receiving a stranger's kidney, who could then donate the kidney to one of thousands of other renal-failure patients, nor would I have to receive a kidney from a cadaver. As it turned out, DeleVan and I are 97% compatible (very high). If you want to know why we were so compatible, you can read *The Cosmic Family, Volume I*—one of the books I authored, in collaboration with several "unseen" friends. DeleVan felt that she came into this world (among other things) to give me one of her kidneys. She was a surprise identical twin who became God's magical gift to me as well as for many others who hear her sing her powerful voice in TaliasVan & The Bright & Morning Star Band, TaliasVan's Bright & Morning Star Choir, and in her own band, VansGuard. [Gabriel of Urantia is also known as TaliasVan & The Bright & Morning Star Band with his music career.]

My daughter DeleVan, the donor, singing and playing keyboards with her band VansGuard

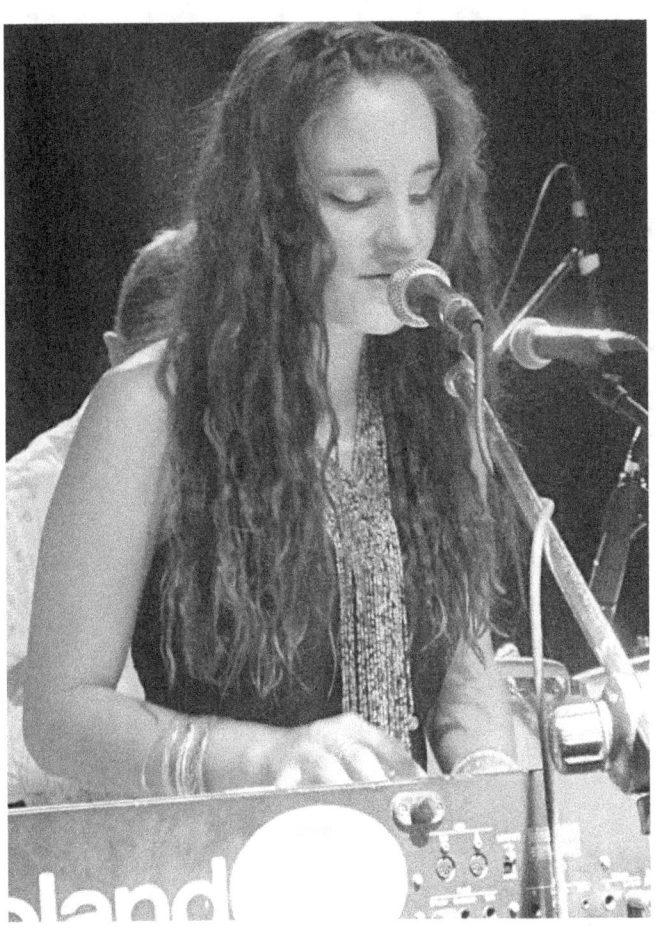

PART 1

THE SHARP END OF THE NEEDLE

(Dealing With Diabetes, Dialysis, Transplant And The Medical Field)

A Series of Journals

Part 1 of this book is a series of journals I wrote during the months of my process, from the time of discovering that my kidneys were failing to the recovery from having a kidney transplant. They were written on the day they are dated, right in the middle of my process of being a patient in the throes of surgery, dialysis, and more surgery. What I write is very honest, raw and real—in the moment of what I was thinking and feeling at the time.

May 2010

Getting Bad News, Wondering, And Wrestling With God

I guess every person who is told that he has an illness that can lead to death goes into a state of shock. I sure did. "God, what have I done wrong?" I fight off self-pity and bitterness. I wonder if God has forsaken me. "What good can come out of this experience?"

I—all of a sudden—spend half the day, three times a week, in dialysis. "Hey, God, is time not important anymore?" I feel disoriented, and my days are segmented.

Foods I loved have been eliminated from my diet. I am told I have a food-eating disorder. "So I guess I deserve this suffering? On this planet can we really enjoy eating? Those 'horrible' French fries! Those 'terrible' sausages!" I hear (again) that most of what I learned to love to eat all my life is wrong. (Of course for many years people had tried to tell me this, including a friend-physician of several years.) Here is the poison list: fried chicken, fried fish sandwiches, fried potatoes, pizza, ice cream—bad, bad, bad! What a planet!

Everywhere I look, I see overweight people on their way to some kind of disease, including some of the doctors, nurses, and aids. "Take me to another planet. Beam me up, Scotty." We all live in delusion for sure. What a joke that I ever considered myself a healer, with a little "h" for sure.

It seems to me that almost everyone has some malfunction in their body. One of the best human beings I ever met died in his sixties of cancer, and he seemed so healthy. He actually beat me in tennis, and, at the time, I was thirty years younger than him.

At times it seems as if very little in life really makes sense on this fallen world. So, where do you go with that realization? Make plans for what? So often we have no control over life. Maybe we are programmed. But by whom? Are we puppets on a cosmic string? Is God so cruel? How does free will fit in? If we are living on a fallen world, is every choice doomed to failure?

How do we make any sense of this?

"OK God, what do You want me to learn? What is the lesson?"

"Shit happens."

"Uh, I thought You were in control of everything. Aren't You omnipresent? Is there anything we, Your children, earn by our service to You and humanity? Are rewards only in heaven? So why not do anything we want to do while here on earth?"

There's that free will question again.

"Hey God, I thought I was making good choices."

Hmm, maybe I did blow it in the eating choices. Karma, karma, karma. Those nasty French fries, fried potatoes, fried chicken, hoagies, pizza—bad, bad, bad! Hey, didn't I bring this up before?

How do people find meaning in lives of daily drudgery? Why are souls trapped in diseased bodies? Why are babies born with horrible rare diseases? These children have to grow through their toddler, preteen, and teenage years with these diseases, trying to make sense of their lives.

Those stricken children with healthy minds try to deal with their abnormal bodies and find some dignity with their peers. Is it bad karma they need to work out? With some maybe, but with others you can see in their eyes a beautiful innocence and courage in the way they deal with their disease. Why does God allow their suffering? I could more easily forgive God for my suffering, but I do not understand the suffering of the innocents.

Both my grandmother and grandfather (basically good and new souls) died peacefully in their sleep. I thought they were blessed. But they were by no means saints. My grandfather particularly was rough around the edges. Why do others have a much more tortuous death than my grandparents?

Some people suffer so much physically in their dying process that they ask for a mercy killing. I think that sometimes makes sense when someone is already in the process of dying anyway. OK, does shortening the dying process (euthanasia) interfere in God's perfect will because the person is to suffer their negative karma? No, I really do not believe God is a masochist.

Hospital Experiences

So, I had just found out, at sixty-three years old, that I had kidney failure, was entered into the hospital through the Emergency Ward at St. Joseph's in Tucson. After some tests I was also told that I had congestive heart failure and needed to have an operation to unclog my heart passages—a double whammy in one day.

A tube was inserted into my leg that went up to my heart to open up my arteries. Then stents were put in to keep those passages open. During this time, a catheter of sorts was also put into my chest so that I could receive immediate dialysis while in the hospital.

When they were done with that operation, off I went to dialysis. I was informed that I could not move my leg that had the tube inserted into it due to the chance of causing something to tear thus I could bleed to death. So I had to lie still for three hours through the heart operation and three and a half more hours of dialysis.

I wanted to scream. I think I did yell at the dialysis technician to allow me to move an inch. He was merciless. The room was freezing, and he still had a fan blowing right on me. He reminded me more of a truck driver than a dialysis technician, in speech and mannerisms. I wanted to pass out but could not.

I asked God what I did wrong to be punished this way. Particularly when I looked around the room and noticed that I was the only person in the dialysis ward under seventy years of age. I suddenly felt old and forsaken by God.

Later, at the dialysis center I was told that I could possibly do home dialysis but needed a fistula in my arm and that meant another operation to put in the fistula.

fis•tu•la (fĭs′che-le)
An abnormal duct or passage resulting from injury, disease, or a congenital disorder that connects an abscess, a cavity, or a hollow organ to the body surface or to another hollow organ.[1]

What I didn't know was that the fistula works by injecting 1" or longer needles into the arm, as an intake/outtake in the arm to cleanse the blood. I thought it worked like a catheter, where you just twist off the tube tops and connect the tubing. But that is not how it works. The fistula is supposed to be a better way of doing dialysis because it cleans the waste out of your blood more effectively. So, as an outpatient I received an operation that attached two main veins to make one large vein.

Only two weeks before I was admitted to the hospital, with almost-dead kidneys I still was able to perform (sing and play guitar) a two-hour concert. I did collapse right after the concert. I thought I was just tired.

I was planning on touring several states in the summer. That was all over. Now dialysis three times a week at a center, half my life taken away by sitting around having dialysis. Endless doctor visits and tests take away the other part of my life. Yet there was hope for a kidney transplant.

The pessimistic East Indian nephrologist assigned to me when I was in the hospital said with my heart condition he doubted I would be considered a candidate for a transplant. Because TiyiEndea and I felt we needed a more hopeful and positive doctor to work with, we got another nephrologist as soon as was possible.

I found out that doctors in private practice have no direct authority structure over them. Patients easily could become another cash-register ring. At a university hospital that was less likely to happen. We met my new primary care doctor and his superior at the same time. My new primary care doctor scheduled me for a colonoscopy test, a major test necessary for any applicant for a kidney transplant. Going up my behind with a long tube camera did not sound too pleasing to me.

The hardest part of this whole colonoscopy was having to drink a gallon of liquid barium, which tastes horrible, even though they add the word "berry" they should have added "scary." I had to do this again several months later when I actually got the kidney transplant.

July 19, 2010

More Ordeals

The test is two days away, and I have to fast on liquids for forty-eight hours previous to the test. I should add that I have to drink a gallon of the worst-tasting liquid you could ever imagine, in order to poop my brains out before the test. Yuk yuk yuk! Nothing like having to take dialysis on an empty stomach. I already feel the dialysis takes all the life force out of me.

Of course the dialysis companies claim the process gives you more energy. The executives should all try it. It could never take the place of a real kidney. It does keep people alive, depending on your definition of what alive is. For me, I can only go through this ordeal with the hope of a kidney transplant so that I can resume my life. I feel so bad for those over seventy who have no hope for a transplant.

July 28, 2010

Money-Driven Medicine

Now I am dealing with medical insurance issues. Sometimes it seems that some of those people working in this system want to make sure that I worry that I might be dropped—kidney transplant or not—dying without a hope of a kidney transplant.

Whether medical coverage is private or public, it seems that patients have to do battle with these companies and systems to get them to cover our care. As a pastor, I have worked with the poor and indigent most of my life and hopefully have helped hundreds of people in their rehabilitation to become contributing, taxpaying citizens. But neither the government nor private medical insurance companies care about my or anyone else's service to humanity or to the country.

I think that the government as well as private companies in the medical field should care about saving and prolonging people's lives, especially those who do contribute to the true progress of humankind, which includes many people who have little or no money for medical care. In the United States, often it seems as if the government cares more for business profit-making interests than it does for the people. At this time, available health care for all of its citizens is just a dream in greedy America.

I have to confess, I am looking forward to the Judgment Day.

The Disease Of Diabetes

Most people do not realize how bad the disease of diabetes is when it is secretly and quietly eating away at your body parts. I was in denial for many years, like many people who do not want to change their eating habits. I probably could have saved my muscles in my legs from deteriorating due to high-sugar levels had I realized I was getting neuropathy. I probably could have prevented the loss of sight in my left eye if I had taken the disease more seriously. Diabetes affects every part of the body, and most people with it do not even know what is happening until it is almost too late.

Diabetes is considered by many in the medical field as the disease of the poor people because a high percentage of these people have it. Many thousands of people with diabetes do not get proper health care due to being underinsured or not insured at all, and so the disease gets worse.

Now, those politicians ruling Congress want to drastically cut back the government's medical programs for the poor. In Arizona, many cuts are being considered, including covering certain specialists like podiatrists. I wonder how many thousands of diabetics will lose their feet because they no longer have medical coverage to see a podiatrist? I pray I do not lose my feet because I cannot afford seeing one.

I have done my own research and now eat much better than in my earlier years. Thank God for my wife, TiyiEndea, who is an excellent caregiver.

I have four children, my youngest daughter being thirteen years old. I noticed after having her, my sexual life began to decrease, and erectile dysfunction became more prevalent. I was in my fifties. For some men when this happens it is the end of their life emotionally and psychologically, because with diabetes even Viagra and other medication for this dysfunction do not work.

Thank God that I have a sense of my own value and a loving wife who sees me for who I am. I think that diabetes is one of the most horrible diseases on the planet, for, as I said before, it eats you up a bit at a time.

I am hoping with a new kidney my sexual life will come back to where it was. Of course it will never be the same as when I was a young man, and getting older is a fact of life.

I have discovered that sex plays a very little part in true love, and obviously my wife has discovered this too. When you really love someone, the spirit of the other person who you want around you and that companionship is the greatest blessing in one's life.

August 1, 2010

Small Victory

I will be transferring to another dialysis center in Tucson where they will begin to poke my fistula to get a buttonhole made. The plan is that while there every day for a month TiyiEndea and I will be trained on the home-dialysis machine. If my fistula works, at some point they will remove the catheter on my chest.

Not having a catheter in my chest will allow me to get in a pool with my whole body and do water therapy. I look forward to this freedom. If all goes well with this plan, until I receive a kidney transplant, I will do home dialysis five days a week for two hours at a time, but at least it will be at home.

August 5, 2010

The big day is coming; a meeting with those who determine if I am eligible for a kidney transplant. My overall tests will help determine that.

August 13, 2010

Eligibility

I was told on August 5 that we can proceed to try to get a kidney transplant, providing all the tests come out according to their standards. We were also told there is no use going to school every day, eight hours a day, for home dialysis if the kidney transplant can be expedited. My medical-coverage plan has not agreed yet to pay for the transplant even if I am accepted for this by the team of doctors.

On one of my uncommon days off from seeing doctors or taking dialysis, I had to go to the lab to get a blood draw for an HIV test. I know I do not have HIV, but it was required anyway, even though there is no final approval for a kidney transplant.

I was denied a pancreas transplant by the head surgeon of the medical institute, even though this could completely heal the diabetes. Even though my heart tests came out above normal, he was concerned about the stents in my heart. I was also told that when in surgery and being under anesthesia so long with both a kidney and pancreas transplant, there is a chance that my heart could not take it. On top of that, for their own reasons, a patient fifty-five or older is too old for a pancreas transplant by their standards.

I know that these concerns for my age would not really matter in my case. I was told by a chiropractor, who practices Chinese bone setting, that my bones were like a twenty-nine-year-old. I had to laugh, because I am always saying to people that I am twenty-nine, and I often feel that young. I do think that this chiropractor was right on the mark in his assessment.

The medical coverage I have will only pay for a pancreas transplant when the kidney is being transplanted at the same time. I guess it is cheaper that way. So if I ever do want a pancreas transplant later on to try to heal the diabetes, my coverage will not pay for it. I do not know where that fits in with the most recent health-care plan that has been adopted by the government for the people of this nation, but I guess I will find out down the road if it is ever possible to get a new pancreas.

The pancreas transplant is also a very expensive operation, and, like millions of other diabetic Americans, I would not be able to pay for it, and my current health-care coverage will not pay for it. So much for the health system! We definitely do need socialized medicine in this country. Of course, I can go to Canada and become a citizen, or England or France or even Cuba—as a matter of fact, just about anywhere in the developed Western world but the United States.

A New Dialysis Center

The new dialysis center, called Fresenius (which designs dialysis machines), is much more professional, and it definitively has a higher sense of being germ-free, even though it is my hope that in a few months I will have my new kidney. In the previous center, which was a DaVita Center, a technician almost killed me with the mistakes made. It reminded me of my first experience in the hospital when I got emergency dialysis after my heart surgery, where the technician was about as sensitive as a rock. I felt like I could have been accidentally killed there too. Both times, TiyiEndea and I were tempted to walk out, but of course, my life depended upon that dialysis I was receiving so we could not do that.

The Donor

My daughter, DeleVan, has been contacted, and she will also go through a series of tests and interviews. Even though there is always a chance that the kidney transplant will not take, there is a higher possibility that it will from a sibling or other relative, who is a living donor, than a kidney from a cadaver.

This dear daughter is a twin, and when she came to this world, she was unexpected because she was not detected by either the doctor or the midwife. I had sensed her presence along with her sister in the womb at least a month before she was born and told the doctor and the midwife that I thought my wife was having twins. But they did not believe it until they saw for themselves after she was born.

More Ponderings

Could it be that DeleVan came to this world to give me her kidney, among other wonderful gifts she has already given me? Time will tell. Why doesn't God just heal my old kidneys? Questions, questions, questions! And some of them it seems God just does not yet answer. Maybe He never will, and I will have to learn to live with those unanswered questions.

The alternative to transplant is the rest of my life on machines, which I cannot fathom. Temporarily I can understand, even write about it to teach other people, but I do not see how the rest of my life on a machine can serve humanity or that a just and loving God would ask this of me, who has given everything I can give since I was twenty-four years old to the service of humanity. (I know, I know—this is a lot of complaining.)

I am not in any way demanding anything from God, but it is expressing my spiritual dilemma, trying to understand and explain the nature of our loving Universal Father. I, along with hundreds of thousands of others over the centuries, have asked the questions. Why do good people suffer? Why do innocent children die or live with terrible illnesses? And so on.

I have noticed many people on dialysis—some very young, but most in their seventies and eighties. It is obvious that many of them are not iniquitous people. Why did their kidneys give out? I think it has more to do with the foods we eat today—the chemicals, processed sugar, and other unhealthy additives. There are always a few who abuse the body by alcohol consumption, but I believe that is a minority. And yes, some do overeat and tax the body, tax the kidneys. People who love life also love to eat and enjoy the taste of food, just like they enjoy other blessings in life.

I once knew a wonderful, kindly man who had been a social worker in his younger years and became a minister in his midlife. He was primarily a vegetarian, did not smoke or drink, and yet he contracted liver cancer. Try to figure that one out. The last thing he said to me, on his deathbed just hours before he passed, was "Keep the faith." He knew I was thinking, "Why did God let this happen to him?" I am sure he was wondering this himself, but with his dying words he was able to overcome his own doubt and keep his own faith, and, up and above that, the concern for my faith. So it seems to me that definitely bad things, in many ways, happen to really good and decent and righteous people.

Back To The Medical Process Of Getting A Kidney Transplant

The head of the nephrologist department of the University of Arizona Medical Center said that I needed to take a stress test. This concerns me. Not that I think that my heart is not strong enough, but that since my hip fracture and neuropathy in my legs, I know my legs are weak. So I do not know how the doctors are going to do this stress test with my weak legs on a treadmill and expect to get a good stress measurement. I am lucky sometimes if I can stand on my feet for any length of time. My legs will give out before my heart will.

I also now have, for the last several years, a limp. I attribute this mostly to the orthopedic doctor who put a rod in my right leg to heal a fracture, knowing that it was going to shorten my right leg possibly an inch. If he would have told me that was going to happen, I definitely would not have agreed on that treatment. I later learned that there was an alternative that would have been better in healing the fracture. Now that it is done, what are they going to do, re-break it? No, I will have to walk with a limp for the rest of my life.

In these journals, I share my own ups and downs with my health and the medical field as I experience them in the moment. I am being honest with my thoughts at the time because I know so many other people have similar struggles and thoughts. If I can honestly share my processes, then hopefully these journals will help someone else get through their ordeals and "keep the faith."

August 23, 2010

Referral To The Podiatrist

I told my primary care doctor—who we saw twice and now he is going to be gone for a month, so we will be seeing his substitute (so much for personal care!)—that my feet and legs hurt, so he referred me to a podiatrist. I could just as easily have gone to a dentist, because all he did was prescribe for me diabetic shoes, which had already been prescribed for me by an orthopedic specialist. This podiatrist also said that I could have surgery for damaged nerves, but that is not guaranteed to help.

He did not even prescribe painkillers for my legs; he referred me back to the primary care doctor to do that. Why he did not do it is beyond me, but I have noticed that most doctors are very careful not to take too much responsibility if they do not have to. You know, liability and lawsuits.

So many doctors play it so safe, which I can understand to a point, but sometimes it seems so impersonal and that the patient is not really a person but a machine in these particular doctors' eyes. With them, it feels like you might as well see a mechanic than a specialist, whatever the ailment is.

Several weeks have gone by now, and I have not heard from my health insurance that they will pay for the expenditure of the special shoes. I guess they will, but by that time, I will probably have to go through a lot more pain in my legs and feet.

Dialysis Administration Lack Of Coordination Between Them And Patients

Now you would think that once you are assigned days and times for dialysis, that this would be kept consistent by the dialysis center, but this does not always seem to not be the case. Why it is not consistent is beyond me. The head nurse the other day said we can no longer come in at our normal 9:30 A.M. slot and changed it to 11:00 A.M., even though we told her it is hard for us to meet other doctors' appointments that same day (which sometimes takes us weeks and months to get). She did not seem to care but reluctantly gave us one last 9:30 A.M. slot.

When we went at 9:30 A.M. the next morning (and we have to go twenty miles one way), that nurse was not there that day, and she forgot to tell the administration office of the time change. We were told that we were down for 11:00 A.M., and then we were informed, "You can just come back tomorrow" (on my day off).

Shuffling elderly dialysis patients around is convenient for the staff but not so convenient for these elderly people, and I am not talking about myself. For those elderly whose only means of transportation to and from is not their caregivers (like in my case my wife). So they miss transportation times with social-provided transportation.

As I was complaining to the office administration of my messed-up situation, there was an elderly person there with no idea of how he was getting back home because his time slot was messed up too, and his transportation had left before he found out that he could not get dialysis that day. In situations like this, it seems that convenience for the people scheduling the slots is more important than the patients and their situations.

There was an elderly man in his early eighties who had been on dialysis for three months, with a catheter, who did not know that the catheter area entry point needed to be kept really clean or else he could die from infection. He was told that he should try to get another access entry point as soon as possible, and get the catheter in him removed. TiyiEndea explained all of this to him because he was confused, and he did not have anyone there to be his advocate.

Yeah, you are given manuals and booklets to read, and sometimes a DVD is provided that explains a lot about your situation and the protocol. But what is an eighty-something-year-old man going to do with reading material or a DVD with no one to assist him personally? He had no family member or friend to help him understand all of this. Nothing beats direct person-to-person communication that complements the reading material. All too often patients get a sense of being mere numbers and slots to fill rather than human beings that need care and consideration.

I am now told how important it is to have the same nurse inject the needles to build a buttonhole for the fistula so that there is consistency with one person. Then after I get my fistula, that nurse said (only after two usages) that she is not going to be there next week and someone else would have to poke me. The problem with that is, if someone else hits a millimeter away from the last entry point, the buttonhole is not going to take so easily. That means I will have to continually get poked in new spots, and I can tell you, those pokes hurt like hell when a 1" needle goes in my arm from two different entry points. Again, so much for administration scheduling and the concern for the patients.

So what happened? My fistula did not work the second time, and now I have to worry about some operation to put what they call a balloon in my fistula, so my blood can flow through my veins faster.

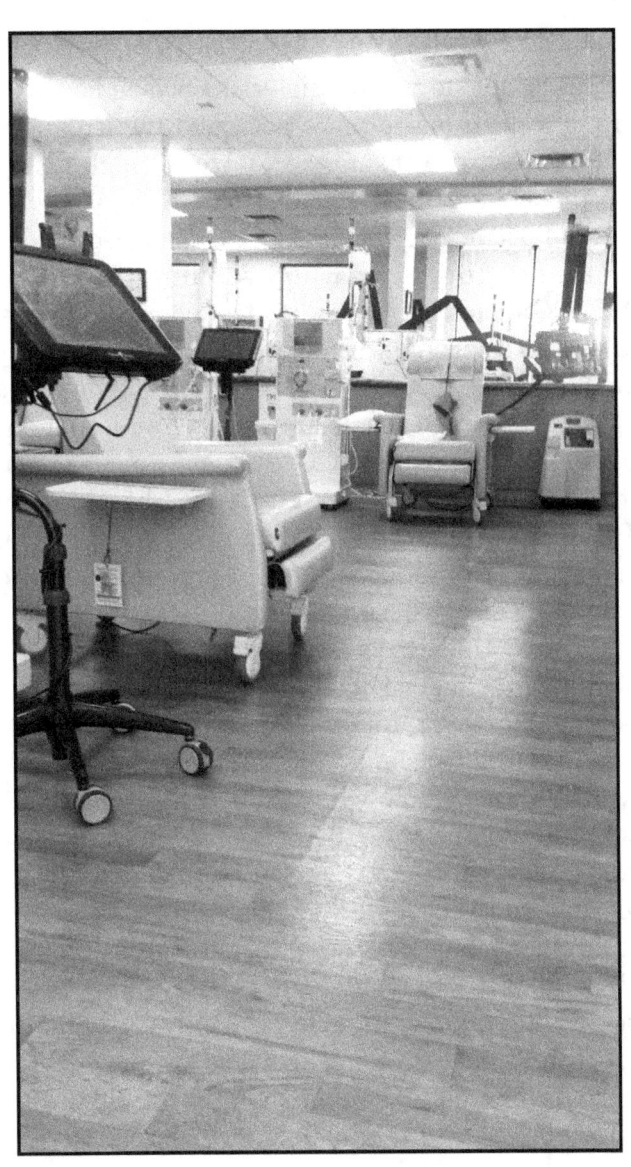

The dialysis chair

Health Insurance Problems

To be able to pay for dialysis, a person has to be either a millionaire or be accepted by private or government-run insurance. Arizona Health Care Cost Containment System (AHCCCS) is Arizona's form of Medicaid, which is a government-provided insurance for those who are poor. To get on AHCCCS a person has to be at an extreme poverty level, and so people who do not qualify because they are just above that level but cannot afford any type of insurance are left uninsured. As a result, millions of people have no medical insurance coverage and thus often do not get much-needed health care. Thousands (maybe tens of thousands) die from serious health problems because they are unable to pay for medical care.

I hope that the newly-adopted nationwide health-care plan can change this situation for most people. However, on this plan, all people will be required to have some kind of medical insurance, which means people who cannot get AHCCCS (or something similar) will still be required to have some kind of coverage. Common sense would dictate that the coverage be on some type of sliding scale where people pay what they can afford, so that all people—poor, middle class, and wealthy—will be able to have some decent health-care plan to cover their and their family's medical needs.

If that is not the case, and some people cannot afford the cost of the insurance, they will have to decide to spend their money on either feeding their family or having medical insurance. Of course most will choose food over insurance, and thus they may be going against the law because they do not have required medical insurance. That will be just one more thing to be stressed about, and stress is a big contributing factor to poor health. Hopefully the system will be set up so that these things do not happen, but I am not going to hold my breath on that one.

    Even if someone has insurance (whether private insurance or a government-run plan like AHCCCS) and needs expensive treatment like dialysis or an operation, often those insurance plans have a protocol to stall treatment. I have heard this over the years from patients as well as from a few people who used to be medical insurance processors. I did hear from two social workers that AHCCCS stalls even certain operations that could determine life or death. In my case I experienced my medical coverage stalling for a kidney transplant operation, even though I had a live kidney donor.

    These medical insurance companies and health-care coverage plans play with people's lives—from the top executives down to the person who supposedly makes the decision whether to provide or not provide coverage for a particular medical need. And patients, whose lives may be on the line, have to grin and take it.

    Power and greed corrupt those who have no sense of themselves nor compassion in their hearts nor an understanding of ethics. You have to wonder why some people can become so callous and cruel working in a field that requires a sense of social responsibility and humanitarianism. Though there are many sensitive, caring, and hard-working people in the health-care fields, there are also some very uncaring, cold, mechanized people.

September 10, 2010

The Sharp End Of The Needle

It hurts like hell when I am poked with the beginning 1" needle in my left arm fistula by incompetent technicians or registered nurses who have a rough touch. I do not always get poked by people like that, and when it is done by a more competent technician or nurse with a gentle touch, the hurt is not as bad.

Until it works properly, I cannot get the catheter taken off my chest, which is a direct link to my heart, which is a direct link to death if it gets infected. So you would think that only properly trained, competent technicians and sensitive nurses would do the insertions into the fistula.

My arm, for several weeks now, has been swollen and aches. The head nurse of the dialysis Fresenius Center seems to miraculously do it right, and she even gave me lidocaine to numb the area. This can be done with a smaller needle before the injection of the 1" needles. I am told that they want to increase the size of the 1" needles in time. I hope by then I have my kidney transplant. We will see.

One of the technicians, who is not a nurse, tried to do the injections first. I was told she knew what she was doing. Instead, she put the two needles too close to each other and caused spasms in my arm and clots. So the head nurse took over, and she injected me four more times in different spots, but because of the spasms and clots, even she could not work a miracle. They could not even do a one-on-one, which means one fistula injection and one catheter line. So they ended up just using the catheter.

Tomorrow I have to go back, knowing that the head nurse will not be there. Maybe I would have better luck with the janitor injecting me. I fear that I am going to go through another ordeal tomorrow without that particular nurse being there. The problem is that the fistula still has to be injected because it will fail permanently if there is not some blood flowing. So I get injected, knowing that it probably will not work. I sometimes think that my arm becomes a test tube for these inexperienced technicians. I hate it.

But I do not have an alternative unless I transfer to another center, where I probably will find another administrative inadequacy happening. I do not think that there are enough really good nurses and technicians. Like good singers, good mechanics, good cooks, good teachers, good politicians, and so on, they are far and few between. When it comes to life and death, this is really bullshit.

Somebody needs to pay more attention in the health fields in the dialysis area and injecting these patients and trying to get the catheters off, so that the patients do not get infected and possibly lose their lives because of the inadequacy of injecting technicians and administrative failure.

I do want to admit that, as terrible as the dialysis is as an experience and the loss of time, it does keep me alive, and I have at least 4 good days a week when my energy level enables me to work and enjoy life to some degree. So, I am very grateful for that.

Good News Has Arrived

A woman from the kidney coordinating committee called my daughter, the donor, first and then two days later they called me. I guess they figured my daughter, DeleVan, would tell me, as they did ask her to ask her father if the date was OK. Like we are going to say "no"? Anyway, DeleVan got back to the woman right away, after talking to TiyiEndea and me, and we confirmed with my daughter's transplant coordinator. We have not yet heard from our coordinator still. TiyiEndea did send an email to our coordinator and my daughter's coordinator, asking them what is going on. Interestingly, it was DeleVan's coordinator who called us two days later.

We have learned in all of this medical bureaucracy that if you do not keep your nose in your own business and push your own buttons, sometimes nothing gets done.

I was informed that on November 9 I will go in for my surgery for a kidney transplant. That means I only have, as of this writing, twelve more days and forty-eight more needle pricks. (I always want lidocaine to numb my arm and then the two larger blood transfer needles, which are now up to over an inch. I think they call the one now a 15-guage.)

To be on dialysis for the rest of my life would be almost unbearable, yet thousands of patients have no other option if they want to live. Some make the best of it and live those four other days to the best of their ability, even working in jobs.

Working is quite possible, because this is my day off of dialysis, and I am writing this. But as far as I am concerned, on the dialysis days the best thing that I can do afterwards is eat and space out, to some degree. My body and mind are not quite together, and my legs tremble. I can hardly stand after a treatment.

Many dialysis patients need to be wheeled out in a wheelchair. Usually they are older (in their seventies) though I have seen some in their forties and thirties and even a couple of people in their twenties, which makes me very sad. I am in my mid-sixties and think I am too young to being doing this dialysis stuff!

I realize that being a layman, I may get certain medical terms mixed up and not sound exactly like a professional medical person, which I am not. I am a patient, telling this from my side of the hospital bed and dialysis chair.

A Sobering Experience

The other day, even though the professionals knew my water weight was to be taken down to a certain number, one new dialysis nurse and a technician failed to take my weight down to the proper number. This causes a number of things to happen and can effect every organ in my body as well as my eye sight. I felt pretty good right afterwards, because not as much was demanded of my body right away, but as the evening went on, I got weaker and weaker and even fell when I tried to walk. I began to have some stomach and chest pains.

I know there are technical reasons for all these symptoms, but again I am not a doctor writing from a doctor's perspective. All I can say is the nurse and technician failed to treat me properly, and the dialysis did not cleanse my blood as it should have that day if I had had the correct water weight.

Many nurses and technicians are quite burnt out from long hours and repetitive work. Many of them are unhappy on the job, and I cannot blame them a bit because most of the patients are on their way to the next life. I guess it is kind of like working in a hospice, except the system tries to keep people alive because dialysis brings in a lot of money.

Again, for someone like me, who has no plans of dying and wants to live, dialysis is a lifesaver. I just wish that they could do it in a much more painless and professional way. The head nurse of my dialysis center is a gem, who knows that her calling is from God, and she is excellent at what she does. When she injects me, I hardly feel any pain, but she is so busy that I do not get her every time. She is a gift to all of us patients, and I think that she is underpaid and overworked.

Nearing the Transplant
More Sobering Experiences

I was told by my nephrologist as well as a nurse in the dialysis center that I should get the flu shot to give me more protection when I receive the transplant. So I went ahead and received the flu shot at the dialysis center. The next day I immediately got sick for about three days. I tossed and turned all night in pain the third night and woke up with slurred speech and a fever. I reluctantly decided to go to the Emergency Room to be checked out. The next two days were a nightmare.

I was kept in the hospital for testing. I had an x-ray, two MRIs (1 for the head and 1 for the neck), and many other tests I cannot pronounce. They told me I had had a slight stroke. I missed my dialysis appointment at the center and was given dialysis there at the hospital. The nurse, who was unfamiliar with my fistula, must have stuck me at least four times and caused clotting and swelling. It hurt like hell, even with the lidocaine that I asked for several times.

The nephrologist in the hospital came in and told me that certain medicines that could cause me another stroke would not be given to me. In the meantime that order did not get on the charts in that hospital, and a nurse came in and gave me the medicine anyway! If my faith was not where it is, well, figure it out. I only pray for God's protection.

To make matters worse, the assistant to the head surgeon who was going to do the transplant, told me they were going to delay the transplant, thinking that it may be a problem with my heart, and that they wanted me to take a cardiology test, even though I had one just a few months back.

The cause of the stroke is unknown, but I think possibly it is a result of two things—the inexperienced technicians from the main dialysis center allowing my pressures to drop so low that I almost fainted and the flu shot. My immune system was just not strong enough to handle all that was being asked of it.

The head nephrologist of the hospital now disagreed with the need for a cardiology test, saying there is nothing the matter with my heart, that the problem was a clotting in my brain stem. So while the doctors are battling, my transplant (as far as I know) is going to be delayed. The head surgeon and the nephrologist have different opinions of why I had the stroke and the need for a cardiology test. They had all the time in the world to give me a test when I was in the hospital, but now that I am out I will have to go back in for that test.

I can hardly believe the inefficiency of even a Magnet, well-maintained hospital with excellent physicians and quality nursing. It seems as though too often the left hand does not know what the right hand is doing, even in a top hospital. I cannot imagine what happens in a lower quality hospital. In my case, the dialysis center is not in communication with the transplant team, even when one of their patients is on the list for transplant.

Official Postponement Of My Transplant

It is official that my transplant date has been postponed another month. Now I am scheduled on December 7.

Enduring one more month of dialysis because I had an Ischemic stroke is hard for me to take. I understand that the transplant team wants to be cautious and observe me for that extra month, even though everything seems OK and my speech is almost back to normal. So, I must take forty-eight additional shots with needles that seem to be feeling bigger each time I get poked. Four additional weeks of sitting in a chair for 4 hours, three days a week, which I hope to become more positive about than I am right now.

Here We Go Again

Ok, now it is back to doing what we had to do at the beginning of all of this process. I need to get a different primary care doctor again because the one at the transplant hospital is always an intern with no experience. Likable enough, but they get transferred, and we have gotten new ones a couple of times already. This will not work for me.

I need a new nephrologist because the nephrologist I have is not connected to the transplanting, though she is connected to the hospital. That is like having a car with motorcycle wheels.

I need a new cardiologist because the one I have now does not "click" with me due to some things I perceive in his character. It is not wise to have a doctor that the patient does not trust.

The only saving grace in all of this is the vascular surgeon, Dr. Leon, who is friendly and concerned enough to spend some time with TiyiEndea and me and answer our questions. He seems to be competent and assured in what he does.

November 12, 2010

I cannot possibly write all the details of all the specialists I have to see again before the transplant, but my life consists of dialysis and doctor visits in between. I dread going to dialysis because Fresenius can't seem to schedule my shift with a nurse who is experienced enough to stick my arm and find my vein through my fistula. God, it hurts. I pray that I can make it another month. I watched several technicians fail to properly stick an Indian woman on her arm graph yesterday. They finally gave up, and she went home and had to come back the next day. She was in a lot of pain in her arm due to the improper sticks. She normally is a cheery person, but not this day.

Oh yeah, I am losing my hair thanks to the medications, and that is not counting the anti-immune medication I will have to take after the transplant. They say it is to keep my body from rejecting the kidney.

I hope my insurance continues to pay for the over $2,000 per month meds. I have heard of poor people dying because the government drops their insurance and they can not continue to pay for the medications and take the pills. I plan on going to a naturopathic M.D. and see what I can substitute for herbal medicines, providing I can afford the herbals, as my insurance provider (and most other insurance companies) do not pay for natural medicines.

November 29, 2010

I saw one naturopathic doctor so far, and he told me that he knows of no substitute alternatives. I will keep looking.

I only have four more dialysis days left until December 7. I have all kinds of fears. One is that the kidney will not take. But I push that aside because my donor, DeleVan, and I are 97% compatible. I am concerned about having another stroke or even getting a bad cold. So I am walking, you might say, on tippy toes with viruses and wear a mask at dialysis.

Some little things I noticed about Fresenius is that they have policies to cover their own butts and beyond. Like they do not want you to snack on anything while on dialysis. Easier said than done when you have to sit there for four hours. So they will not let you even heat a cup of coffee in the microwave (if you can sneak one in). The head nurse, as good as she is, also chose the policy over another technician helping me to take my laptop off my lap, correcting the technician for doing so. It looks as though Fresenius puts policy over patients.

The place is clean enough, but when I got dialysis in Nogales at DaVita, the technicians actually sang while they worked. I never saw that in Fresenius. And a few times DaVita passed around donuts and other snacks to the patients. It was a much warmer atmosphere, although maybe not as healthy, eating sugar donuts. But many of the patients, who felt they were dying anyway, did not care and enjoyed the donuts.

More Thoughts On The Real Causes Of Disease

One thing that I have learned from this experience, from watching the Native American people on dialysis (for many from the reservation come here), is that bad things happen to good people. I do believe that people manifest certain diseases, but these people that I have talked to here were victims, as I feel I have been a victim—a victim to others' wrong choices, not always wrong choices of my own.

Non-actualization of destiny is the greatest cause of diabetes. Many people who eat terribly and are obese never lose their kidneys. Others do, because of diabetes and stress. But non-actualization does not help anything.

These people "live lives of quiet desperation," (to quote Henry David Thoreau). They cannot afford proper education and live lives of poverty or near poverty. I am sure they too have dreams that they have to put aside to just survive. I see it in their torn faces—the suffering, the desperation, the hopelessness. I heard one patient say he would rather die than have to continue on dialysis.

Everyone does not have the hope of a transplant, although transplants are becoming more accessible. If you are over sixty-five, you will not receive a transplant, even though people are living longer today. I just made it by the skin of my teeth. My mother is eighty-two years old and still kicking. She has diabetes but still has all her limbs and organs.

There was a time when my sugars were up to 700, and I tried to deny that I even had diabetes. I thought that I was just going through a temporary stage. So I did not take care of myself or pay much attention to the sugars. I chose not to take insulin and get the sugars down. I did not realize that the high sugars were eating muscles in my legs and my organs, particularly my kidneys. Who knows? If I would have been higher in my actualization of my destiny and traveling and making music, I could have eaten those foods and have those foods not bother me, like they do not bother a lot of simple new souls who are obese but quite content and happy. It is a paradox.

I do know that I will have to be more aware with the new kidney of what I eat, and I will do that, for I never want to have to take dialysis again. I think I would choose the option of home dialysis. It will take training of others and my wife for six hours a day, five days a week. The treatments will have to be everyday at home after the training. My wife will have to do the sticking. I pray we do not have to do this and the new kidney will work.

I do know that I have also a genetic disposition to diabetes and that my pancreas needs to heal. I believe I will heal my pancreas completely and beat the diabetes, not to affect my new kidney and pancreas. But it isn't just eating that affects the organs, which I wrote about in another book, called *Teachings On Healing, From A Spiritual*

Perspective. You see, on a fallen world we are affected by the choices of others more than we think.

Recollections Of Past Traumas

Like I said previously, I tried to deny (when I was younger) the diabetes. Several years ago I was sitting at my desk, going through a lot of stress because someone I was dealing with could have affected negatively all of the people I love if, instead of a lower choice, he would have made a higher decision. But as it was at that time, he was not going to make that higher decision. All I can say is that through this stress, sitting at my desk at that moment, I lost the sight in my left eye. The eye doctor I saw blamed it on a stroke, and the optic nerve was destroyed in the left eye. This led to a series of laser treatments to the right eye, as the right eye was bleeding from retina disease due to the diabetes.

Later on in 2011 I had to go back to a specialist eye doctor in Green Valley, Arizona, and this woman on several occasions put 1-inch needles in my eye. After going back several times and sitting in the overcrowded waiting room and hearing one elderly man mentioning this treatment never helped him, I decided to get up then and leave and explore other avenues of healing. To this day, my good eye still bleeds, and I have to receive some laser treatments to stop the bleeding.

I had already developed what is called neuropathy in the legs, because of the high sugars. But I have to say, again, that if I would have been in my higher actualization of destiny, I do not think the sugars would have affected my body as much as they have.

One evening, when I was getting out of bed, I fell, hitting the doorway going from the bathroom to the bedroom, fractured my hip, and was rushed to the hospital. The orthopedic surgeon put a titanium rod in my right leg, never telling me I had a choice of letting it heal naturally and never telling me that the operation would shorten my leg (which was already slightly shorter than the other one, from birth). This increased shortness due to the operation causes me to walk with a limp and limits my exercise and walking.

The reason I am writing this all in a book is because life happens and so do unexpected traumas. As Confucius said, "Always expect the unexpected." People have to learn to live with a lot of things as they age, that they do not even think about when they are younger. I thank God that I have access to a pool that does provide me the means of getting some exercise. I know that even with my new kidney, I have to walk more, and I intend to do that.

I have to overcome my fear of losing the good eye I have. To this day, I am still getting laser surgery on my right eye, due to macular degeneration—a disease that diabetics are more susceptible to. There is nothing I can do about the short leg. I do not want to refracture my hip to remove the rod. That will be with me for the rest of my life.

December 28, 2010

The Transplant — December 7, 2010

I remember being wheeled into the operating room, but I do not even remember being given the anesthesia. When I woke up, which seemed like seconds later, I was told that surgery was over and that I had my new transplant. Wow! Celestial Overcontrol must have taken me somewhere while I was "under" during the operation. I remember having many visions of past lives, mostly on battlefields.

For a while after I woke up from surgery, every time I closed my eyes, visions of other lives came. I saw more with my eyes closed than open, so I kept them closed. I was under morphine, and I am sure the drugs actually accentuated the experience, but it definitely was an experience.

Having my daughter's 22-year-old kidney that was working very well caused me to need to pee right away. That was a great sign that all was working well. As a matter of fact, every half hour I had to pee. Then came all the drugs and the immuno-suppressants. Damn it, I am losing more hair! Oh well, vanity oh vanity, always vanity.

I was in the hospital about five days, which was record time. Thank God, no more dialysis. My last dialysis was on Monday, December 6, one day before the operation, and wouldn't you know it, they had to stick me a couple times before it took. Please God, never again!

I fully intend on starting some sort of dialysis chaplaincy program for all those patients who have spiritual questions as to why this is happening to them and little or no hope and truly no advocacy, because the dialysis centers are profit-making organizations, with many owned by doctors who are not really trying too hard to get people off of dialysis.

I, along with TiyiEndea, was my own advocate. We had to push even the transplant coordinator to follow through. And we did. We wrote letters, made phone calls, sent e-mails, and did it all. As a result, I got my transplant in eight months, which is record time.

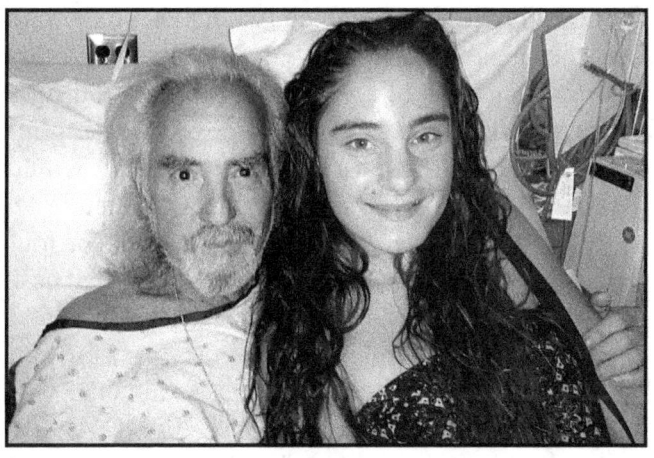

**Right after transplant
Dad and daughter, DeleVan**

Remember the East Indian DaVita nephrologist who said I wouldn't be able to get a transplant? I will send him an e-mail telling him I received my transplant on December 7. HA-HA.

One thing I have learned, when you have to do it all yourself and be your own advocate, hopefully you find another one within the system. So I want to begin by thanking all of the transplant team of the University of Arizona Medical Center in Tucson, Arizona, starting from Dr. Rainer Gruessner, Dr. Kaplan, Dr. Kasturi Ranga, Robert Diana, Annette Whinery, and the whole transplant team, with the exception of the social worker. All she wanted to do was hand us papers.

My only complaint is that the transplant team has no endocrinologist, which is a diabetes expert, to keep the sugar levels even. We've been getting cross information from others on the staff, including a pharmacologist, and my sugar levels are higher because of the drugs. You would think they would have an endocrinologist on the transplant team.

So now I have to go back twice a week for four weeks, for blood tests and meet with the staff. These little pricks are nothing like the dialysis pricks, and I don't have to leave long needles in my arm for four hours. It's a prick, and you're done. Thank God. In a few weeks I'll only have to go once a week. And so far everything is going well. I'm healing at the incision and the black-and-blueness is going away, as well as the pain.

I couldn't taste my food for a while, but some of my taste is coming back now. All in all, I feel like I have a new lease on life and hope to sing and play guitar in the May 2011 festival and then continue to do concerts.

There are many things about the bureaucracy in the medical system that really need to be revamped, mostly the left hand not knowing what the right hand is doing. But thank God for the technology and for the doctors and technicians who have the minds to serve humanity in this wonderful transplant process. They are really special people, and I thank God for them. Even the dialysis nurses and technicians—who have a lousy job to do—kept me alive until I could receive a new kidney. I wouldn't want their job.

One nurse told me that the needle pricks always work best when there is some kind of relationship between the patient and nurse or technician. I know that they are overworked, and they can't be in too much of a hurry or else they will hurt the patient and miss the vein. So for any nurse who reads this, I pray you take your time, know who you're poking with that needle, and realize that without the grace of God, this could be you.

Post-Dialysis Syndrome (PDS)

I noticed that I have had a sense of anxiety and a feeling of being trapped. I'm naming it "Post-Dialysis Syndrome" (PDS). I had to pray about this, and what I heard from God was that it was because I sat in a chair for four hours a day, having to keep my fistula arm with the needle injections still all of those four hours, three days a week. If I moved it

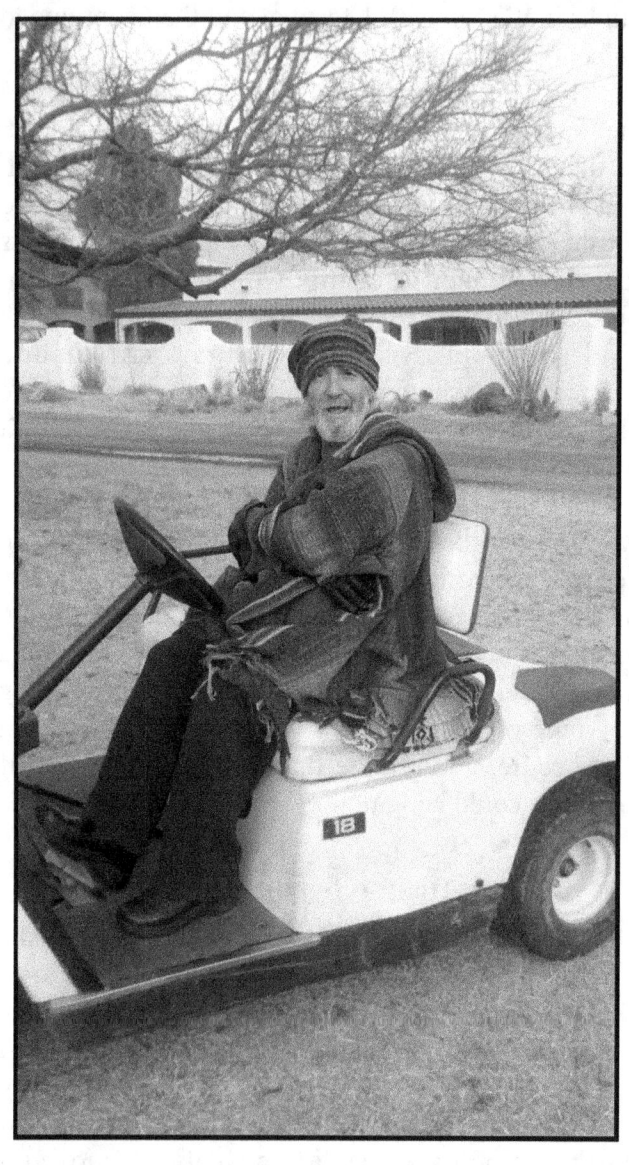

First day out at the ranch after transplant

slightly, the machine would start screaming and a technician would have to come. So only my right hand was available to scratch my nose, use the laptop, or whatever. I was exactly trapped for that time. It's hard now to feel that I'm free. There is always the concern of losing my kidney. But I feel as time goes on I'll gain more faith and confidence that I'll be OK and that this kidney will last me the rest of my life.

January 12, 2011

I sent letters to the following persons, to try to get a chaplaincy program established at the various Tucson, Arizona dialysis centers, but no one replied to this offer from our church to provide chaplains for their patients.

Fresenius Medical Care
1. Julie Joseph, Area Manager
2. a nephrologist who has part ownership in Fresenius Medical Care

DaVita Tucson Dialysis
1. Ken Futch, Regional Director (Regional Offices)

February 22, 2011

My Daughter's Post-Transplant Care From The Transplant Team

On February 15 the donor (my daughter DeleVan) along with my wife TiyiEndea (who drove her) went to the University of Arizona Medical Center's Emergency center because DeleVan was bleeding very heavily on her period, thus we were concerned that she was hemorrhaging. One of the transplant team's coordinators and doctor's assistant—knowing that my daughter had an unhealed incision and was having problems with it—denied my daughter admission and did not consider it an emergency. The transplant team knew my daughter's incision was not right when 3 doctors touched it and saw it on her regular check-up visit in January 2011 to the clinic. She never received a call back to look at it and has to wait until March 2011 for her next routine appointment. I pray that it is nothing serious and nothing is going on inside that should not be going on. You would think that her hemorrhaging big clots and her going to the Emergency Ward would prompt the transplant team to look at her now.

While in the Emergency Ward on February 15, my wife and my daughter sat there six and a half hours before they were told that the hospital just went to Code Purple and had no rooms left. Even though my daughter was a transplant donor patient of that medical center, she was not treated with any special attention. The staff there treated what they considered more "emergency" situations like people with cuts as a result of fighting, alcoholics, and drug users. They never really looked at my daughter—a kidney transplant donor.

After being told that the University of Arizona Medical Center had no more rooms open, TiyiEndea and DeleVan went to Tucson Medical Center, where they had to wait another six and a half hours—thirteen hours total in Emergency Wards. My wife and daughter had to stay overnight in Tucson in a motel, incurring more expenses.

I hope that at her routine March 2011 appointment date, DeleVan is not told that her incision needs to be re-opened to correct something, which would mean another stay in the hospital for her and more trauma.

My Post-Transplant Care From The Transplant Team

Our biggest problem was with the pharmaceutical coordinator, who was less than helpful with us having to deal with getting all the immunosuppressants on time and clueing us in of what was expected of us from the apothecary, because there is a lot of red tape, and, if you do not call them in advance, you have to wait three days to get the pills or medications. When your life depends upon these medications to live, that is really very poor professionalism and could cause a person to lose his new kidney. Because we were not given adequate information to assist us in this, we had to drive a two-hour round trip three days later to pick up the medications. Thank God we had three more pills left!

The apothecary also needed a doctor's authorization or the pharmaceutical coordinator's authorization, which we had not been told about. You would think the pharmaceutical coordinator would know that. Why is it that we had to learn everything through trial and error, when the transplant team, and particularly the pharmaceutical coordinator, is supposed to be there for us? This is not the case with our situation.

I am very thankful that I have a new lease on life and that the surgeons, head neurologist, and other transplant doctors do their jobs efficiently. But often the lower realm of transplant coordinators and assistants seem to not cooperate as efficiently with each other and with their patients. There definitely needs to be a lower-management supervisor to oversee people at this level at the University of Arizona Medical Center and probably at other hospitals. Post-transplant care is very important, as many patients do lose their new kidneys in the first three months.

I mentioned earlier the need for an endocrinologist on the transplant team, as my sugars seem to be higher from taking the immunosuppressants. After about six weeks, the transplant team finally referred me to an endocrinologist. Guess what? He was right down the hall, and we had to wait another month for an appointment! Why he isn't actually on the transplant team when most of the people who lose kidneys have diabetes is beyond me.

My feet and legs have been hurting more since I have been taking the immunosuppressants. This is due, I am sure, to the increased sugars. The endocrinologist prescribed different insulin and more frequent usage. So far, the new treatment is not working.

Regardless of some of the shortcomings of the transplant team at the University of Arizona Medical Center, I am grateful to them for my second chance at life and deeply respect the fine work that the doctors at higher levels are doing. I talk about the many negative experiences I have had with the hopes that the University of Arizona Medical Center will change these things as well as to warn other patients of the problems if the hospital does not change these things. I hope that from sharing my own experience, other patients can ask the right questions and get things done without going through the hassle my wife, daughter, and I all did.

The following is a letter I wrote to Arizona Governor Jan Brewer asking her to not cut the medical budget to the University of Arizona Medical Center and AHCCCS patients.

LETTER TO ARIZONA GOVERNOR JAN BREWER

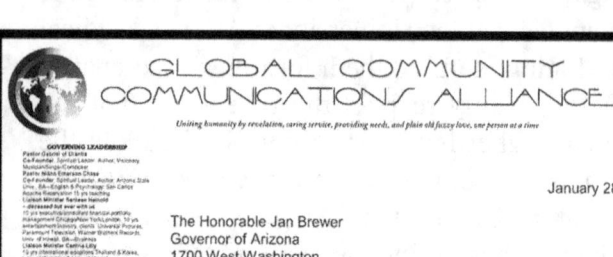

(Sorry you might need to use a magnifying glass due to the size of the book.)

March 7, 2011

Today was my last visit to the University of Arizona Medical Center clinic on a bi-weekly basis. I will not have to go back for three months. I started out, post-operation, going twice a week for two months and then once every two weeks for a month. I have to see my nephrologist at another location every few months too.

With the exception of my high sugars, caused by the immunosuppressants (which in turn causes my legs and feet to have sharp pains and tingling), I feel fine. Most likely the damage done to my feet and legs is nerve damage, caused by the once high sugars from diabetes. I will continue to seek healing for this problem.

Neuropathy affects thousands of individuals with diabetes. Many of them lose limbs, particularly legs and feet. Although I have pain, podiatrists say my feet look good—no sores or redness, which sometimes turns purple.

The biggest problem I have is walking with a limp, which throws my whole body out of alignment and causes discomfort. As I have mentioned before, this is because when I fell and fractured my hip, the surgeon in Cottonwood, Arizona operated and used a hip screw and side plate combination, which caused my leg to be shorter. As of this date, he has not responded to my letters, questions, and concerns.

3 Types Of Dialysis

1. Catheter dialysis — which is two tubes going to the heart. This is a temporary process until you can get the fistula or peritoneal dialysis.

2. Peritoneal dialysis — uses an abdominal catheter in the stomach lining.

3. Fistula dialysis — AV (arteriovenous) fistulas are created by a vascular surgeon who joins an artery and a vein together, usually in the arm.

(Home dialysis is available with different methods through the fistula or peritoneal dialysis)

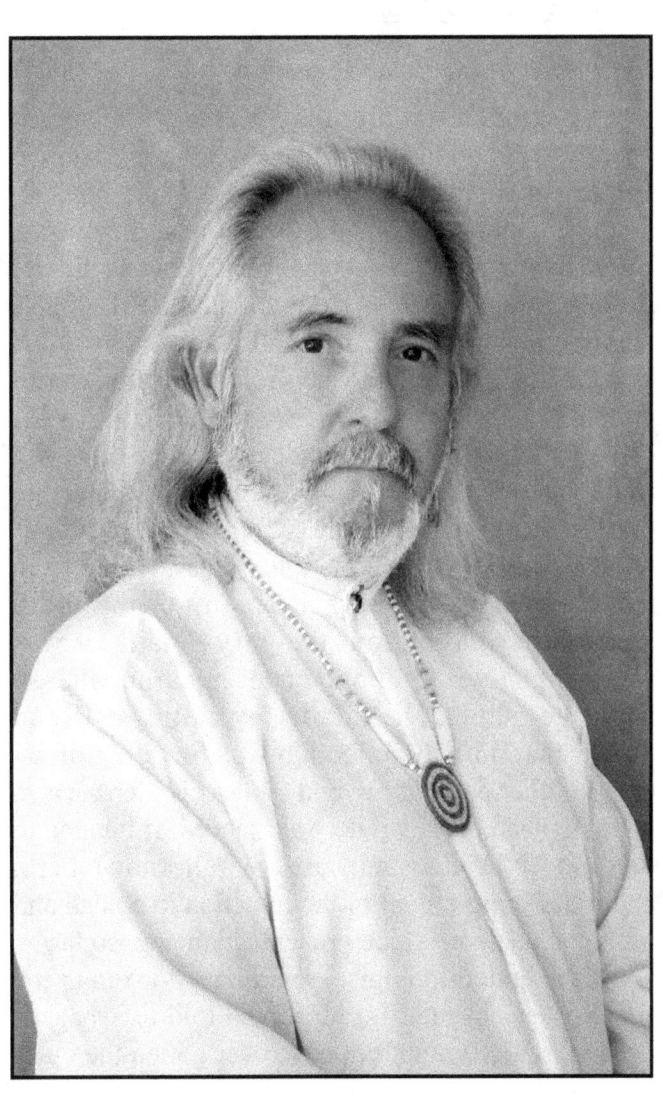

Thanking God no more dialysis!

October 28, 2011

Post Operation

It has been ten months since my transplant operation. I started having abscesses on my arms in September (in the eighth month). I told the endocrinologist about them when I went to visit him at the University of Arizona Medical Center, but he did not seem very concerned. He even said, "Ah, that's nothing to worry about." When I got the second one I called his office again, and probing his nurse with questions, she told us that we really had to start cleaning the area that we injected with insulin with alcohol before the shot. That was a revelation that no one seemed to tell us before.

Unfortunately from the other areas, which were not cleaned by alcohol, I began getting more abscesses. Leaving out the gory details, it was sickening. Then I got one under my arm, where I never got shots. I found out by calling a friend doctor that now the infection was traveling on its own to other parts of my body. Yuck! Under the arm is not a place that I would want lanced, if it came to that. So TiyiEndea and I used a well-known herb, and it did bring out all of the infection to a head and broke on its own, which prevented lancing, so far.

If the endocrinologist would have looked at the first abscess in the first place and told us what we needed to do, I might not have ever gotten the other ones and may not have had to go back into the hospital for two days because here's what happened.

On October 22, 2011, I started vomiting and got a 102 fever. To add to this, my neuropathy pain was worse, and I could hardly walk. My whole body felt terrible. Under the advice of my nephrologist, I went to the Emergency Ward at the University of Arizona Medical Center and was admitted, because any fever is dangerous for a kidney transplant patient.

I was admitted to bring the fever down and hopefully find out why I had the fever or if I had an infection. I already knew I had an infection, because of the abscesses, but they somehow did not relate this to the fever. I went in at 10 o'clock in the morning. I laid on a gurney for fifteen hours, sick and with a fever and moaning, while they:

- took two different sets of blood draws. (Oh those needles!)
- another shot in my stomach, with a needle that looked like it would work really well with a hippopotamus. It was to thin my blood.
- took a head and chest x-ray.
- did a C.A.T. scan.
- did a sonogram of my kidneys for 45 minutes.
- put me on a heart monitor.

And when I got to the next holding area (because I was never really admitted to a real room), they gave me an IV drip, which they should have done in the E. R. for those fifteen hours.

Most of us know that the world is falling apart, but if you want to know for sure, go to the hospital and be admitted. In the E. R. holding room there was no bathroom of course. This room was very small and had no windows, and this would be where I would stay for the next fifteen hours!

And then, after fifteen hours in that room, when I was moved to the next room that they called the C.D.U. (Clinical Decision Unit) section, I still had no private bathroom. Out in the hall was one bathroom for God knows how many patients! So I used a urinal bottle and prayed that I did not have to do anything else, as I was too sick still to walk to the bathroom.

At least I had a more comfortable bed than the plywood I was laying on before. With the exception of the two nurses coming in at 5 o'clock in the morning and waking me up to check my vitals, I got a pretty good night's sleep that night. The two nurses on that floor that evening were really very nice, particularly the head nurse, who I will call Molly. She was a grandmother type and very attentive. So was her helper—not as nourishing but much different than the nurses in the E. R., who were methodical to a fault. All head no heart, with the exception of the two older nurses in the E. R. who were more experienced and allowed themselves to have heart. But it seems there is nothing they can do either, because of the hospital procedures, written—I think—before Columbus came to America.

I mentioned earlier that all too often the right hand does not seem to know what the left hand is doing in the hospital. You would think that there would be some level of management that looked out for the patients rather than the doctors' or administrators' pride.

There was a situation that I was downright dumbfounded about. A nephrologist assigned to me in the hospital (not my regular nephrologist) looked at me the next day—after my fever had broken and I was feeling better. He looked at all the tests except for the last blood test, as they were looking for a certain virus, and, said that I was free to be discharged. TiyiEndea and I exchanged glances, and our eyes lit up. It was like escaping from hell! Before leaving, he smiled, and asked me if I felt like I could leave. I tried to hold back my enthusiasm and said solemnly, "Yes, I think I could do this,"— instead of saying to him what I really wanted to say, "I can't wait to get the hell out of here!"

After a wait of more than an hour, the nurses finally came in and said they had the release from the nephrologist, but now they would need another release from the internal medicine specialist, who had eight floors with patients to check out besides ours. So they did not know for sure what order he was checking them out in and when he would be there to sign my release papers. In other words, even though the one doctor said I could leave at around two in the afternoon, it might be 2:00 A.M. before I actually left, when the other doctor gave his approval. We asked if they couldn't just call this doctor and tell him that the nephrologist said I could be discharged? The day nurse said, "Oh no, we can never do that. We have to wait until he comes on this floor." So I said, "What about all the people who are waiting for this bed and room in the E.R., like I had to wait for fifteen hours?" And she said, "I'm sorry, this is hospital policy." Well, I do not know if that is true or not, or is it the rule of the other doctor's pride?

October 31, 2011

There is a TV series called "The Boss" where the boss leaves his executive offices and goes and works at the lowest of levels for a day or more to know what it is like. I think hospital administrators need to be admitted to the E.R. I have a feeling that this just isn't a problem at this particular hospital or hospitals in general; I think it is a problem everywhere, as more and more administrators lose contact with the common folk, starting from the President of the United States, the Congress, the Governors, the Mayors—most of them have lost touch with the common people.

It is no longer "We the people;" it is "We the Bureaucracy," "We the Corporation." Unfortunately a hospital is a corporation, a big business. I thank God for those nurses, who have to work under these conditions who know what it should be like themselves and are really trying to help people. Many of them become callused and lose sight of the benevolent reasons they first became a nurse. So too do many doctors.

It is not a pleasant feeling for me to continue to have to take the immunosuppressant drugs that leave me with no immune system. And at the same time, I do thank God for the doctors who enabled me to receive this kidney transplant. I pray to God often that no germs or bacteria get a hold of me that would cause me to lose my kidney. By faith, I am expecting the kidney to last well into my much older age.

When we got home, TiyiEndea and I called the University of Arizona Medical Center and were told by my primary physician's office that in order to get another endocrinologist, I would have to actually go see the previous endocrinologist to get his permission. We thought this was more than ludicrous; this was outright insane. So I said, "OK, I will see a doctor from the outside."

I was required to first see my primary physician at the University of Arizona Medical Center, which I did. He found me an endocrinologist not connected with that medical center, and we drove the sixty miles one way to go see her, only to find out that she did not want to treat me. She suggested we go back to the University of Arizona Medical Center, for they have all the case studies on me and computer links to each other.

We wondered why she could not have told me this before we drove the sixty miles. The University of Arizona Medical Center had made the appointment with her office and faxed her office all the information on me. I think she decided at the last minute that she did not want to take a chance on a kidney transplant patient. It would not look good for her if I lost my kidney under her care.

When we got home from there, I called my primary doctor's office back to try to get another endocrinologist at the University of Arizona

Medical Center. That was about four days ago. As of this date I have not heard back from them. (By the way, an endocrinologist is a doctor who specializes in sugar control and trying to keep the sugar levels down.)

I do not think that the head doctors on the kidney transplant team know all this nonsense is going on, particularly the surgeon who gave me the transplant. The question would be, why give a patient a transplant if his post-care is less than adequate? Go figure.

This song was written by the author—who is also
a singer, songwriter, and musician—on October 25, 2010.

The Sharp End Of The Needle

Twelve sticks a week, twelve hours in the chair.
The Devil thinks he's got me for life.
It's almost too much for even Van to bear.
Each day at the sharp end of the needle.

But my daughter DeleVan heard my painful cry.
And offered her vital organ, so I won't have to die.
Or be stuck to the machine while my blood flows by.
Bracing myself for the sharp end of the needle.

Now I don't think it's anything I've done wrong.
I've lived my life to sing His gentle song.
If so many significant others would only have come along.
To walk in His will and try to be spiritually strong.
I wouldn't have to feel the sharp end of the needle. (3 TIMES)

I've felt too much sadness from those who could have helped along
   the way.
That it ate my body and melted the clay away.
If they only would have tried to obey, or even taken the time to pray.
I know I could have avoided the sharp end of the needle. (4 TIMES)

And I don't blame the good Lord not one bit at all.
For He saw the outcome of rebellion's downfall.
He planned to send my daughter long before even one wrong choice.
That Van's clan can forever sing and abundantly rejoice. (2 TIMES)
That I no longer have to feel, the sharp end of the needle. (3 TIMES)

© 2010 Global Community Communications Alliance
All rights administered by Global Change Multi-Media, P.O. Box 1613, Tubac, AZ 85646.
All Rights Reserved.

Experiencing The Aftermath Of The January 8, 2011 Shooting Of Gabrielle Giffords

I felt very connected to the terrible tragic shooting [on January 8, 2011 in Tucson, Arizona outside a local grocery store] of Congresswoman Gabrielle Giffords because of several factors. One, Dr. Rayle—who at the time was a physician for Soulistic Hospice, which I co-founded—was one of the people in the parking lot who was shot at, played dead, assisted in holding down the shooter who had been tackled by someone else, and attended to some of the shot victims before the ambulances came. Secondly, Congresswoman Giffords was taken to the University of Arizona Medical Center in Tucson, where I had my kidney transplant and was going twice per week for blood tests and other doctors' checkups. It just so happened that I had one of these checkups the Monday following the Saturday shooting.

We got there at the entrance at approximately 7:00 A.M., and it took us a half hour to get to the parking area, because of the heavy presence of the media. It was a madhouse. I never saw so much media in one place at one time, and they seemed to be in control; not the police. There were local, state, national, and international media. Their vehicles blocked the hospital entrance and everything else. There was not a policeman in sight, except when we went inside (and I will explain later). TiyiEndea usually drove me to the front door and then parked the car, but we could not get past the media traffic jam, and many other handicapped people could also not get past and had to park in the parking lot and be taken by wheelchair to the front door.

The media was double-parking and also going into the patients' parking lot with unmarked vans. I know this because I saw them coming out of the vans with cameras. TiyiEndea even yelled at one of the double-parkers to move their car so that patients could get by. When we got inside it was mayhem. There was a long line of patients who had now to be checked because the police were concerned about a conspiracy and possibly other shooters trying to still get to Gabrielle.

When we finally got to the front information desk (which took another thirty minutes), we were asked for identification, which we never carry into the hospital and usually just walk right in. I told the young woman that I was a kidney transplant patient and a minister, but she did not seem to care. (I think that she was probably a secretary for the hospital and not with the police authorities or security.) So my wife had to go out to the car and get our identification. They gave us name tags, and we went in. It would have been nice if the hospital would have called all of us patients to inform us of what we needed to get in. I wrote the Administration two complaint letters. A secretary to the C.E.O. did apologize for our inconvenience.

The next time I went to the University of Arizona Medical Center, which was two days later, you would think because we had official name tags we would not have to go through the security ordeal again, but, wrong, we did. At this point I said it would have been nice if this much concern for Gabrielle Giffords would have been taken before she was shot, not after the fact.

I agree with Pima County Sheriff Dupnik, who suggested that political "vitriol," particularly by conservatives, was partially responsible for this and other violent acts against innocent people. He called Arizona "a mecca for prejudice and bigotry." I have lived in Arizona for twenty-seven years now, and Arizona seems to be very behind the times, especially with the right-wing thinkers.

When I lived in Sedona, Arizona, I was aware that Senator John McCain owned property in nearby Page Springs. In many of his political ads he was staged standing near Cathedral Rock in Sedona, implying that his property was right there, which it was not. But I did live near the beautiful Cathedral Rock in the Red Rock Crossing area and fought very hard for many years against the building of a major bridge over Oak Creek there.

The main local A.M. radio station in Sedona had politically conservative owners who provided rhetoric and programs supporting their views, including having a bridge in the Red Rock Crossing area. The major local Sedona newspaper also was owned by publishers with extremely politically conservative views that also supported a bridge near Cathedral Rock. At times, I could hardly believe the things I heard and read from this radio station and newspaper. For example, there was much "talk" against universal health care and against protection of the environment. I believe that due to my more politically liberal stance for health care for all people and protection of the environment (especially preventing a bridge near Cathedral Rock that would compromise the fragility of that ecosystem), both of these organizations and their owners misrepresented me in their media, which they tended to do with anyone who represented views opposite of theirs.

I now live at Avalon Organic Gardens & EcoVillage (which I co-founded) in a county by the border where there is a substantial number of residents who lean politically more towards right-wing, conservatism. The new law SB 1070 that was passed by Arizona Governor Jan Brewer was supported mostly by the Tea Party of Arizona and other right-wingers. So in my particular area, where I co-founded the nonprofit Global Family Legal Services—which specializes in low-cost services for legal immigration—I am not very well liked by some.

I have written much on why there is the separation of consciousness between political conservatives (right-wingers) and political liberals (left-wingers). If you want to read more you can purchase *The Divine New Order* or *The Cosmic Family, Volumes I and II*. There definitely is a consciousness-divide, because the majority of people on the planet and in America are brand new souls, while a smaller contingent are older souls who have been around the astral block a few times.

The day before Gabrielle Giffords' release from the University of Arizona Medical Center, I had to go again to the hospital for a checkup. Most of the media were gone—moving on to Texas where she was being transferred for medical rehabilitation. Police were gone, and so were the wet-behind-their-ears deputized interrogators, so we walked right in, thinking "Hey this is great!" What we did not know was that there was a backup of patients—many who had left when all that other stuff was going on—assigned to come this day. And to top it off, some of the doctors decided to take the day off. It seems that the patients were their last concern. So when we got up to the clinic, we sat there for 3½ hours, and then we were finally brought into where we were to meet a doctor, but he never showed up during the additional twenty minutes we waited for him before TiyiEndea and I decided to leave for the other appointment we had that day in Tucson.

Keep in mind now that I am a recent kidney transplant patient! A thousand and one things could go wrong, and I could lose my kidney and my life. So when they tell you how great it is at the University of Arizona Medical Center and how well they did (which I think is indeed the case) for Gabrielle Giffords and the other victims of that tragedy, they possibly overlooked about one thousand other patients, who would like to tell their story. So I am telling it for them. And you know, many of them are the poor.

One woman, whose husband was a patient who had just died, came with her son and another family member, and guess what? She too did not have her ID when they were doing all this interrogation, so she was not allowed in. People do not seem to bring ID into the hospital. They leave it in the car. I have observed that many of the poor do not even drive; they are transported to the hospital by family or shuttle service.

Well, Gabrielle Giffords is gone now. But what will remain for a long time is the catering to the rich (not particularly Gabrielle Giffords) over the poor, catering to the insured over the underinsured or uninsured, and the incompetent administration and bureaucracy of many hospitals. Long live Patch Adams, whose staff of doctors and nurses work for nothing by donation, to serve the poor, free of charge.

Oh, by the way, I do not know who implemented this (probably the hospitals), but did you know there is a small charge ($3.40) for every AHCCCS patient every time you come into the hospital or doctor's office? So if you go twice per week, that's $6.80, and a lot of poor people, with various kinds of illnesses, need to get blood checks often. So if you are on Social Security or welfare and you have to still spend $7 or more a week, that is one less loaf of bread or a second-hand shirt for your kid. You get the point. This is the real "sharp end of the needle" when the government and the rich continue to stick it to the poor!

Journals Continued

February 2, 2012

Gall Bladder Operation

On Wednesday, January 25, 2012, I went again into the University of Arizona Medical Center for another operation. This time it was for removal of my gall bladder. Do not let anyone ever try to convince you that this is an easy operation. It is intrusive to the stomach. Four projection points have to be made (like a cross) including my belly button, in which probes went in, to suck out my gall bladder by liposuction. They had to blow up my stomach with air, and after the operation when I awoke, I felt just as bad as (if not worse than) the kidney transplant. But the major problems were in post-surgery.

Prior to the operation the surgeon sent me to a cardiologist at the University of Arizona Medical Center who had to clear my heart for the operation. She had my complete medications record. By coincidence, I had an appointment with my kidney transplant team there that week. And they went over my medications again. I also saw my nephrologist that week, who again checked all my blood tests and medications. As part of the pre-op procedures, I had to see the anesthesiologist, who again wanted to know all about my medications.

On January 25, the day of the operation, the surgeon who did the operation, head nurses, and other nurses and doctors had my medication chart and all agreed and signed that this was correct. But after the operation, when I was put into a holding room in trauma (and oh boy! more needles, including an I.V. in the hand at pre-op, from which my hand swelled up), they did not seem to be able to find my medication records! This is not a good thing when four departments cannot communicate with each other and keep updated files on their computers, and when they lose the actual papers, right before pre-surgery. So they did not know what dose of immunosuppressants to give me. Finally they came in with 500 milligrams, when I was supposed to be taking 250.

The point of all this is, supposedly without the immunosuppressants I would have kidney failure. They of course (because they didn't have my latest records on their computers), also did not know what amount of insulin to give me and what kind. I was told by the anesthesiologist nurse, "Oh, not to worry. You will have all those records right there." So TiyiEndea, who knew that my life was in danger, had to act like a hound dog so that I could get my proper medications and on time. Then the nurses resent my wife (who is my main caretaker), and egos get in the way.

On the whole, most all of the nurses are very nice. It is the system that is broken down. When you see four doctors all working in the same hospital and the left hand does not know what the right hand is doing, something is the matter. A computer is only as efficient as the operator who puts the information in it.

After talking it over with some medical people at the University of Arizona Medical Center, they felt that the surgeon who removed the gall bladder should have seen to it that the medication chart was there post-surgery through the computer, even if the papers would have gotten lost.

I probably should have stayed three days, maybe longer, but no way was I going to stay in a situation or a system that is not functioning 100%. So after a day and half, when I was asked how I felt, I said, "Oh great!" I just wanted to get out of there. So they released me. I do not think there was much they could have done for me anyway.

The pain in my stomach was terrible. And to top it off, I had a deep congestion and cough. First I was constipated for several days, and then I got diarrhea—all in the same week after the operation. But gradually my stomach began to feel better as the air and gas were released. But to this date, the deep congestion in my lungs is still there. They said that I needed to walk and walk and walk some more to get rid of this congestion, but when you have neuropathy and a limp, walking is not that easy. They did give me a little breathing machine that loosens the congestion as you blow into it and inhale/exhale.

I did go back to the University of Arizona Medical Center trauma center a week later on Tuesday January 31, 2012 and was seen by a very efficient surgeon who had the reports on my gall bladder that was taken, and he confirmed that it was chronic and had gall stones and it was best that it was removed. He said that the anesthesia often lingers and causes nausea—the reason for my loss of appetite. In these ten days I lost one pound per day.

He felt my stomach and looked at the projection points and thought that all was healing well. I was glad that I did not have to go back into the hospital.

"THE END" (I hope)

DeleVan's Experience As The Donor

When I heard that my father needed a kidney, there was no doubt in me that I would give him one of mine. Interestingly enough, I would not have even known this was possible if not for seeing the movie *My Sister's Keeper*, a month before, where a young woman needs a kidney from her sister. Seeing this movie fascinated me—the idea that an organ from one body could go into another body and keep it alive! It is such a beautiful and miraculous thing.

It was not easy watching my father go through dialysis and see his life-force be sucked from him every time he had to sit hours at one of these machines. This was a very trying time in our lives, particularly for him, and the hope that he would be getting a new kidney soon made it bearable.

It was in May of 2010 that I decided to give my father one of my kidneys. I had to go through very extensive testing to make sure that I was a compatible and suitable donor. This included months of blood tests, urine tests, full body scans, physiological and psychological testing, etc.

It was a faith test indeed throughout the entire process. I did not know if I would be compatible with my father or not. I was tested in spirit too, for I had to also be very private and not share this process with anyone, as it was a personal matter. Yet through it all I knew it was God's will and that it would be fine.

In September of 2010 I found out that I was indeed compatible with my father and that we matched 98 percent! This is a very rare percentage and the doctors were extremely pleased. I discovered that the higher the match the less likely my father's body would reject my kidney. I was so relieved to find this out. The surgery was scheduled for November 7, 2010.

About two weeks before the November 7 surgery date, my father had a stroke. We were then told that he needed to wait for the surgery, and so the date was moved to December 7, 2010. This was hard because we were was so close, and now we had to wait even longer.

That last month flew by though and on December 7 we underwent surgery. We were in two rooms, across the hall from one another. I remember being given anesthesia, but I do not remember conking out. Yet I did conk out and did not awaken until after it was all done! My surgeon (who uses a robot) was Dr. Galvani and Robert Diana pulled my kidney out with his hands and did the stitching up.

I was lucky to be one of the first in the country to go through the single-incision method. This is a small two-inch scar vertical down from my belly button. Otherwise I would have two scars, five and seven inches long. They incorporated my belly button in the incision since it is already a "scar" and so in reality it was a three inch incision.

When I woke up from the surgery I remember seeing a very bright blue light. It was magical and ethereal. I honestly did not know where I was or why, but I thought that maybe I had passed on! I was very out of it. The light was so beautiful and emanated a very peaceful feeling. I thought I might be seeing something from the "other side." I was in such a deep, deep state of consciousness that coming out of it into the reality and atmosphere of this world felt almost painful and disconcerting.

I remember seeing the face of a man I did not know. He was wearing scrubs and was hovering over me. He kept touching my face, stroking my hair, gently grabbing my arms, and speaking to me. He said, "Come on back, sweetie," and "you are my hero. Do you know that? Everyone, come meet this lovely hero!"

I remembered why I was here and what went on and felt like I was slowly coming back into my body. This nurse's name was Kelly, and he was an incredibly comforting spirit for me. He was so genuine, sweet, and loving. I really felt blessed to have him as the one who took care of me right after my surgery.

I then saw my mother. She told me that my father was fine and doing very well. I think I may have cried, and if I didn't, I felt like it. I was so overjoyed that everything went well. Though I wanted to express this I really couldn't. I was still so foggy and in a drunken state from the anesthesia.

I was rolled into my hospital room, which I shared with another woman. There was curtain between us for privacy. She had the TV on for most of all the night, so this made it a little uncomfortable, particularly for my minister friend, MaritaSeen, who was staying with me and caretaking me.

MaritaSeen was asked by my family to be my caretaker post-surgery, and she really did a wonderful job. I was so blessed to have her presence near me. She massaged me, bathed me, fed me, made sure I was comfortable, called the nurses for me, etc. She also slept on a chair for four nights in the hospital! She was a blessing.

The pain was excruciating, I have to say. The doctors told me it would be uncomfortable, and they were not joking! But I was given morphine to maintain the pain. Because my stomach was filled up with gas (so that the surgeons could get around my other organs to reach my kidney), after the surgery all the gas has to escape the body. It traveled up into my shoulders and neck and ached and ached.

In spite of my physical pain, those first couple of days after the surgery I was in an extremely peaceful state. I have never felt this peaceful in my life, and to be honest, I felt closer to the celestial beings all around me than I ever have. It was a very spiritual experience. I felt a calm that embraced my soul and washed over me in gentle tides.

Initially I was given a catheter because I could not pee yet. My kidney was in a bit of shock and had to start working again. Unfortunately they took the catheter out too soon and told me "drink up" and I bloated up like a pregnant woman and could NOT pee no matter how hard I tried. It really hurt because my bladder was about to explode! We called the nurses and they came and drained my bladder.

Then they had to put another catheter in. When cleaning my "you know what" with iodine I experienced a new kind of pain. I am not sure if they put on too much iodine or if this is something that happens, but I burned and burned "down yonder" terribly! In fact, all I could do was silently cry. Simultaneously they forgot to give me my dose of morphine and were half an hour late. So that entire half hour I was in tremendous pain. My stepmother, TiyiEndea, made sure they came into the room pronto to give me some morphine, and an extra dose while you're at it, thank you very much.

That experience was the only thing that stands out in my mind as an unfortunate incident. The rest of my time at the University of Arizona Medical Center was very lovely, and the staff was helpful, caring, and attentive.

A couple days after the surgery, I walked with my mother to the room where my father was staying (a few doors down). I remember the feeling inside my heart when I saw him. I was overjoyed and emotional. I saw in his eyes that his life-force was back. They were sparkling and alive, full of life! Seeing this in my father's eyes made every discomfort and ounce of pain from the surgery worth it a thousand times over. My heart overflowed with happiness to see this in him.

I was really very blessed by this entire experience. It was the most fulfilling thing I have done in my life thus far. To know that the quality of my father's life is much improved by my left kidney in his body is a beautiful thing.

I am so grateful to my mother, Niánn, and stepmother TiyiEndea, for all of their love and support throughout this entire process, and to MaritaSeen for being an amazing caretaker. But most of all I want to thank God who has created us and knows the beginning from the end.

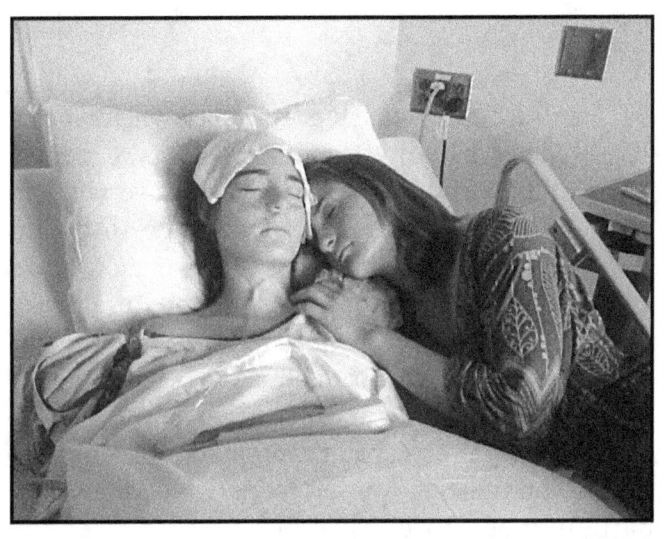

**DeleVan, with her twin sister
SanSkritA, recovering after surgery**

Appeal For More Organ Transplant Research And Artificial Organ Transplants

This chapter resumes with the author, Gabriel of Urantia, continuing on with his story.

There are many young people born with diabetes Type 1. They inherit it from their parents' genetics. Many of these children lose a kidney at a very young age—some as teenagers—and have to go on dialysis. The following is a story of a young teenage girl I met in post-surgery at the hospital. I use a fake name for her, for privacy reasons, but she is one of perhaps hundreds, maybe thousands.

I first met Angie and her mother at the post-operation, organ-transplant waiting room, then again in the blood-testing waiting room, which transplant patients need to go to twice a week after the transplant. It is a one-poke process and nothing like dialysis, but it is hard to get away from those needles!

Angie told us she received her kidney from her mother a week after my transplant from my daughter. Angie was cheerful and quite mature and intelligent. Her mother told my wife and me that Angie was born with spina bifida.

> Spina bifida (Latin: "split spine") is a developmental birth defect caused by the incomplete closure of the embryonic neural tube. Some vertebrae overlying the spinal cord are not fully formed and remain unfused and open. If the opening is large enough, this allows a portion of the spinal cord to protrude through the

opening in the bones. There may or may not be a fluid-filled sac surrounding the spinal cord. Other neural tube defects include anencephaly, a condition in which the portion of the neural tube which will become the cerebrum does not close, and encephalocele, which results when other parts of the brain remain unfused.[1]

Her mother said Angie has had twenty-seven different operations, and she is now nineteen. She had been on dialysis for four and a half years before she could receive a transplant of her mother's kidney, because Angie had other complications. I questioned her, "I would like to ask you a spiritual question. Did you get mad at God for all you have been through?" And her answer was, "God does not allow more than you can handle."

She was an inspiration for me, because during my eight-month dialysis experience, I had bouts with self-pity and questioning God as to why. I, of course, kept the faith, even though I did not understand what I was going through. Despite my sometimes poor eating habits, there are plenty of obese people who have kept their kidneys and eat much worse than I do. So to me, it is a mystery.

Angie has tubes coming from her bladder and bowel and has to clean her own eliminations herself every day. You would never know, looking at her and talking to her, that she has to go through this ordeal.

Angie is also an inspiration to me because for the rest of my life, I will think of her whenever anything happens to me that I think should not be happening and catch my tongue and my thoughts as quickly as possible to not allow myself to go into self-pity. Angie is studying hotel management and hopes to learn Italian and go to Italy and run a hotel. I know she is in God's hand.

Final Journals

March 27, 2012

Being a missionary in the United States since I was twenty-four years old, more than forty-two years ago, I have earned not enough money, according to Social Security to receive a Social Security check. I lived basically by being given room and board by the church or ministry I was working for. So I did not earn enough points to receive a Social Security check. However, with a new program that started and I applied for, I was eligible to receive a small check (less than $500/month) that I started to receive just a few months ago.

I also became eligible at this time for Medicare. This really opened up a whole new can of worms when it came to picking up my immunosuppressant drugs and other drugs at Safeway, which I had just transferred to from Walgreens because Walgreens no longer carried my other supplementary insurance.

When TiyiEndea went to Safeway to pick up my medicine, she was told that I not only had to co-pay now for these drugs, but that I could not get them because of technicalities that Medicare asked for. And, because of all the meds I am taking, the co-pay would cost $130 to $150 a month. So much for my recent social security checks giving much assistance in paying for other basic needs! When this kind of thing happens to people who have to survive totally on their social security check, how can they live?

It is forty miles round trip to Safeway, and my wife had to drive there at least four times before they finally got all of the paperwork correct so that she could actually pick up my medicine. Each of those times she was rejected, even though several times the automatic voice machine (when she called about this before she left to pick them up) said everything was fine now and that my prescriptions could be picked up.

TiyiEndea said there were elderly people standing in line with the same kinds of rejections. There were people in wheelchairs, and she sensed a general feeling of despair among these elderly people. Many of them have paid into the system all of their lives and now have to deal with the bureaucracy of a Medicare system that does not work as efficiently as it should after all of the years it has been in existence.

When my wife told those working in the pharmacy at Safeway that she was running out of immunosuppressants, which keep me alive, they said there was nothing that they could do! They blamed it on my nephrologist who did not send them the right information. However, we never had any problem before with my other insurance company, and we never had to co-pay for the immunosuppressants, just certain doctor visits, who were specialists. I struggled with this too, that government bureaucracy always seems to have a way to rip off the poor patient.

Anyway, after a few days, when TiyiEndea called again about the availability of my medicine, the automated voice again said the prescription was now ready. When she drove there to pick up the meds, she was told that the immunosuppressants were denied. At this point my wife was fit to be tied and again stated, "So you are saying just let my husband die?!!" The clerk said, "Just a minute," and went to speak with the pharmacist who came out and said, "Well, we will give you just enough for a couple of days. We hope you can get it all worked out by then."

It was nice that they were giving me three more days to live! So she drove twenty miles back home and in those three days finally my nephrologist's office got them the information they needed for Medicare. When she went back, and got my immunosuppressants, she asked for my prescription of insulin. They said no, they couldn't do that, that it's two more days for the approved time. So she had to go back forty more miles round trip and come back in two days, forty more miles (that's eighty miles at close to $5/gallon of gasoline). What in God's name are the administrators of Medicare doing in their "service" to humanity?

It is not a great feeling to know that your life is in the hands of a mistake on a computer through an inept bureaucracy or a clerk working for a corporation that is only concerned about profits. This is the state of our present healthcare system.

To read more about Spiritualution[SM] teachings and to find out what you can do to change the system, go to: spiritualution.org

May 25, 2012

Recently I went back to my nephrologist for a visit. There she told me she wanted me to see a dermatologist (which I mentioned earlier in this book, because a lot of people on immunosuppressants get skin cancer). Then she said she wanted me to get a bone density test, and I would receive some radiation as a result of the test. This is because immunosuppressant patients sometimes begin to have bone loss (osteoporosis).

Doctors are pressured by the medical field to have their patients see specialist doctors and have to cover their own behinds, because if something happens on their watch it is not good for them. This is both good and bad for the patient—bad when you have to see so many doctors unnecessarily. And good of course if there is really something wrong with you. But you would think the patient would know that something is wrong with them first in most cases, like "Oops, I got a lesion here, and I don't know what it is" or "Oh, my bones just feel tired lately." And "If the Viagra doesn't work, I guess it's time to see a real 'bone' doctor. HA HA!"

The fact that no one told me that the immunosuppressants could cause bone loss flipped me out, because from the beginning no one told me that it was another side effect of immunosuppressants. I signed a lot of release forms and probably on page 1,999 at the bottom, in small print, it may have said that. But what is the use of seeing all these doctors if not one of them can tell you that? Are they so specialized that they cannot be informative human beings, informative doctors, just giving you information about their area of expertise because they are afraid, so afraid, of being sued or pissing off one of their colleagues (because their colleague should have told me)? Are they afraid that people would make the choice to die instead of taking these pills, and the drug administration cannot make the money they do? At least Dr. Kaplan (Transplant Team at University of Arizona Medical Center) answered my question in my last visit, when I asked him, "Can I live without these immunosuppressants?" He said that some people do. At least that gives me a little hope for when this whole economic system fails. And that might be sooner than we think.

June 13, 2012

Near-Death Experience

On Thursday, June 7, 2012, I went to a dental appointment with an alternative dental practice. This was my second visit there. In my first visit I got a deep cleaning, and afterwards I felt a little dizzy and turned white in my face. Even some of the staff there noticed it and asked if I was OK. I thought I was, so I did not think anything more about it. I just attributed it to the pain that you go through with teeth cleansing.

On the second visit, this time the hygienist again said she was going to use some gel to numb the area, as she had to go deep into the gums to clean them.

(Diabetes helps to deteriorate the gums, which causes gingivitis and periodontal disease and the loss of teeth.) I guess we did not ask enough questions in the beginning, and the dental staff did not provide a meeting with us to explain just why they are "alternative." As of this writing, I still do not know exactly why they are "alternative," because what she used was lidocaine—a drug commonly used in the dental and medical fields. This time not only did I immediately feel dizzy, but I felt a tingling all throughout my body and started getting hot. So I sat up, trying to gain my equilibrium. The next thing I remembered—approximately twenty-four hours later—is waking up in the critical-care unit of a hospital, thinking that just a short time had passed, maybe an hour or so.

    This is what my wife TiyiEndea told me actually happened. When I passed out at the dental office, the hygienist pulled me back into the chair, where I then had an anaphylactic allergic-reaction seizure and proceeded to throw up. I vomited all over myself and lost all that good spaghetti that I should not have eaten in the first place (which shows, after all I have been through, how stubborn we humans can be when we crave something). The dental office immediately called the ambulance service because they could not find a pulse. My wife and 14-year-old daughter, of course, went ballistic. I do not know where I was, but I was not there. I understand that it took the ambulance (which was about five minutes away) 20 to 25 minutes to get there.

    The poor dental staff did everything they could before the ambulance got there—some things right and some things they shouldn't have done (like turn me on my back with my head back). I understand now that they should have turned me on my side so that my food still in me wouldn't be aspirated into my lungs. However I'm sure that this was a shocking experience for all of their staff, who are very kind and professional people and probably had nothing like this happen to them before. Leave it to me to be a first in many areas!

When the ambulance came, the hygienist had enough sense to tell the paramedics, "You might want to take a sample of what I used to the hospital." One of them said, "Nah, we don't need it," and she did not insist. But the paramedics should have taken it, as that information possibly could have saved my life. The paramedics also said they did not think I was going to make it to the hospital, so they decided to take me to the nearest hospital, which was St. Mary's. I do not think the paramedics should have said that to my wife, with my 14-year-old daughter close by who could have overheard it. My wife also said that when the paramedics finally got to the dentist's office, they seemed to move very slowly, as well as slowly driving to St. Mary's. I guess they really thought I was a goner, but they should not have assumed that.

My wife, who was in a state of shock, does not recall everything that the ambulance service may have done to me in the ambulance van or in the trauma room because they would not let her in. She remembers that when I came out of the ambulance I was tied down with straps on my arms and wrists and that they also put a needle in my right shin because they could not find a vein with enough blood pressure.

When I got to the Emergency Entrance, they put other straps on me because I was shaking and flailing from the discomfort of all the invasive apparatus they had put in my body. They also put a catheter in my penis for twenty-two of the twenty-four hours. I was strapped down all that time too.

A very kind woman in her forties from the Tucson Fire Department crisis and trauma division was there at St. Mary's to support my 14-year-old daughter shortly after the ambulance arrived.

I do not know what happened there in the trauma room, but I was told by my wife (who was there with me in the background) that because I aspirated my lunch while throwing up, they had to put a breathing tube down my throat to help my lungs breath and expand. Once I was stable, the nurse placed a second smaller tube alongside the first larger tube, but this one went into the stomach to suction out any remaining food. One benefit from the breathing tube expanding my lungs was that it loosened the thick congestion that had been in my lungs for months, which I am still coughing up a week later. That is a good thing, although it is uncomfortable.

Five minutes after I got to the trauma room, my wife went in anyway and watched from behind a screen and got as close as she could. She saw that I was really struggling for them to get the tubes out of my throat, as it seemed that I could not breathe and I was hurting. They saw this as a good sign that my body was still functioning and my reflexes were reacting. At one point in the trauma room there were fifteen people working on me. I was told by my daughter (when I got home from the hospital) that my wife was yelling out in shock to my soul not to leave her or my family or church and that I was needed by all. I do not remember any of this.

From the tubes being in my throat, when I did awaken twenty-four hours later in Critical Care, there was an excruciating pain every time I swallowed, and even now, a week later, I feel pain in my throat. The hospital staff said it would go away in a few days, but it didn't. When I was in the hospital no one looked at my throat to see how bad it was. It could have even had gotten infected. So when I got home, I had a doctor friend look at my throat, and it was very blistered. Sometimes you have to be your own advocate in any hospital and say what you think they should do.

At some point (I don't know when) in the trauma room, the medical team thought I was stabilized, they allowed my 23-year-old twin daughters and my 21-year-old son to come in, as well as my 14-year-old daughter. Stabilized means I had a consistent heartbeat and "okay" blood pressure. But all of my family went through this trauma, as families do when they think they are going to lose a loved one. This was especially hard on my one twin daughter, DeleVan, who gave me one of her kidneys a year and half before.

A nurse practitioner was probably the worst experience I had while in the hospital, for she was prideful and acted "put out" and unfriendly around my wife and even me. When a nurse (who was from Africa) had the sensitivity and efficiency to take a culture of my congestion (because I was coughing up golf-ball-sized mucus), the practitioner, when asked by the African nurse if she wanted to have it tested, said no. I saw this as a power-play on the nurse practitioner's part, as she should have responded in a higher way to the more efficient nurse who was caring for me through the night. I was told by TiyiEndea that this same nurse practitioner also gave her a hard time in the trauma room when she had questions, acting like "Who are you to ask these questions?"—even though all over St. Mary's Hospital in every room it says on the bulletin boards "It's OK to ask questions."

Being a spiritual man, I felt comfortable in St. Mary's, which was originally founded by a group of Catholic nuns. Even though the hospital was recently bought by Carondelet, it still has the name St. Mary's along with Carondelet. There is a lot of religious art and crosses in most of the rooms and hallways, and there is an original beautiful chapel from the 1890s that has the Stations of the Cross, which reflect the suffering of Christ that probably lessens the psychological suffering of the patients who see it. St. Mary's has been known for helping the poor and underprivileged since its inception in the 1890s. And because many of the staff are still Catholic and have a faith, they seemed to be kinder in my experience, even than at University of Arizona Medical Center. Even the doctor, Dr. Michael R. Kretzer, said "Blessings to you" when he left me. He also was in tune enough to see that, with my progress of recovery in two short nights, he could release me to go home, knowing that I would heal better at home and get more sleep, which is a major problem in any hospital.

Here are some of the problems I experienced.

1. When in Critical Care—where a lot of people never get a chance to go back home but die instead—being very sensitive, I felt the energies of despair and death. A woman directly across from me was in terrible suffering. She died that evening. In reality, this elderly woman—in my opinion—should not have been kept alive and plugged into all those machines. They should have unplugged her and let her go home and die in peace.

Part of the problem I think with the medical industry is that they try to squeeze every dollar out of the insurance companies that they can, and the poor nurses who work there have to put up with that abusive system. That is why they lose a lot of nurses to work in hospice or more healing environments. This is why you need to read Patch Adam's article in the back of this book.

When they moved me to the regular patient ward, one woman kept crying out, "Somebody help me!" all night. She was in some kind of horrible pain it seems. When these people cry out, I think a lot of the nurses think they are crying out because of physical pain. That may be part of it, but I think they are also crying out because of the emotional pain that life has dealt them. I think this patient was eventually sedated, but it was not until almost daylight. Another woman just had one of her legs cut off from the knee down, and she was in shock.

2. I had two IVs in my right arm attached to an IV machine, which pumped water into me. They came in every so often and took blood. Even though they took blood in the trauma room, they had to continue doing it every so often to make sure certain internal functions are doing O.K. And since I am a kidney transplant patient, there is always the concern of losing the kidney. This IV machine sounded like a large clock at night and then an extra buzz every so often, which no one as sensitive as me could sleep.

3. The bed was a hospital bed, automated to buzz if I got up, because they considered me a fall possibility and needed to come in to walk me to the bathroom. So even when I tried to pee in the portable urine bottle by sitting on the side of the bed, the bed would go off.

4. There would always be buzzes with other patients calling for the nurses. Even I had to buzz them once or twice and had to listen to my own buzz until they came. These loud electronic buzzes make it impossible for people to sleep. And I often wondered why they do not have a lighting system—you know, like flashing red lights that go off at the nurses' station. I am sure they could come up with something better than the loud buzzes.

5. Another thing that kept me awake was knowing that my wife tried to sleep beside me in the reclining chairs that most hospitals give spouses when they stay overnight. My wife stays with me

whenever I'm in the hospital overnight, for as long as I'm there, and they always give these reclining chairs that are bulky and have a hump in them and are not comfortable at all.

Now in my opinion, the hospital would fare much better if they would use a simple cot (straight) that the spouses could be more comfortable on and the hospital would be able to fold them up easily and store them away. The hospital is always saying how "It's hard to get a reclining chair, but we'll try." That's because the chairs are so big and clumsy. They can easily acquire thousands of army surplus cots for almost nothing from any of the military. Who knows, the hospitals might even be able to get them donated. Anyway it's very difficult for any spouse to know that their loved one is uncomfortable on a reclining chair that doesn't really recline next to them and make into a real, flat bed. Plus, the spouse can't sleep in the patient's bed because the bed will buzz. As a matter of fact, my wife couldn't even sit on it and comfort me. God forbid if any spouse could sit on their loved one's bed and hold their hand!

6. The staff had to come in every so often and check for vitals and poke me in the thumb to test my blood sugar, poke me in the arm to draw several vials of blood to test my blood, and test my blood pressure, temperature, and so on. This is standard operating procedure in hospitals. My arm was so poked that the last time they did it, they had to use my hand. This hurt like hell. Even the nurse said, "If I can't get it the first time, I won't try it again for

now." She did do it the first time, and when she got done, she said, "Thank you God." I said that to myself silently, but I should have said it out loud, and then we would have said it together!

If I ever do lose my kidney again, I am going to look for another Dr. Kevorkian because I am not going to go back on dialysis. I do not want any more needles. More research needs to be done for better ways to keep a person alive while awaiting a new kidney rather than dialysis with blood transference through a machine. They are actually experimenting now on the idea of mechanical kidneys for transplant.

All in all, I feel that St. Mary's staff probably did save my life, although I know that it was not God's timing for me to be "taken" and that He has more work for me to do for humanity on this planet. But it was a close call, probably just what I needed to try to eat a balanced diet. I will probably never eat meat again, at least that is my goal. Not just our physical bodies become addicted to certain foods but our minds become addicted, so we are psychologically addicted. For example, I could have done without the spaghetti that day, but I went to that Italian restaurant because the friendly owners from Italy remind me of my family back in Pittsburgh growing up, even though they probably think I am just another customer.

The woman who lost a leg due to diabetes is one of thousands who eat the wrong food for all kinds of wrong reasons, trying to overcome their emotional pain that life has dealt them, finding some comfort in food. You would think that many of the people who work in the hospital would be slim and trim, but that is not the case. Some of them are definitely diabetes patients of the future. America's greatest problem right now is obesity, even with our youth. I suggest you see a four-part video called The Weight of the Nation. It is an excellent study and very informative. But even seeing this wonderful documentary—which I had my whole community look at—I still ordered spaghetti that day, because of the psychological addiction.

Spaghetti was not the reason I went into a seizure. Do you remember when I said earlier in this book that I took lidocaine to numb the area in which they put these larger needles in me for four hours right before the dialysis? Well, it seems now that my body did not want any more lidocaine, particularly when it comes by way of the gums and goes right up to the brain. My body said "that's enough," and it shut down.

Your Lesson To Learn

The lesson to learn for anyone who reads this book is that if you think you are not allergic to something (particularly lidocaine), it does not mean that you aren't right now, because if you have taken a lot of it over a period of time (no matter what part of the body), taking it one more time could cause the same thing to happen to you that happened to me. So, from now on, when I have any major work done in a dental office, it will have to be a dental office that can put me out with gas/anesthesia.

I hope that this is truly my last journal entry, because I am going to do everything I can do— that I have learned through my experiences—to never ever have to go back to the hospital again.

June 18, 2012

It was confirmed today by Dr. Logan, my nephrologist who ordered the bone density test, that I have osteoporosis in my left hip, femur, and spine. It is a degenerative disease that happens to some people as they get older, particularly people with diabetes and people who do not exercise much. The immunosuppressants accelerate the disease. So, though they help to keep your body from rejecting the kidney, immunosuppressants can create bone disease. Medicine really has to come up with something better for the replacement of vital organs. I am not a scientist, but I would think probably that stem cell research would have the answer to growing a kidney that would not be rejected by the body, because the kidney would be of the body.

June 20, 2012

I have a dermatologist yet to see, to check to see if I have any skin cancer (which is also a possible side effect of immunosuppressants, as mentioned earlier in the book), as well as a neurologist, to see if any of my nerves were damaged by the seizure in coordination with my hands and feet, and a urologist, who will have to test for testosterone levels, which actually help in the strengthening of bone tissue. However, I have to print this book sometime, so you are going to have to wait until the next edition, if you want to know the results.

The point of this book is to hopefully prevent you from going through any of what I went through because diabetes can be prevented and/or controlled, particularly diabetes Type 2—by healthier, balanced, and conscious eating and exercise—and you will not have to see any of the doctors on the next page, that I have listed.

TYPES OF DOCTORS I ROUTINELY SEE AS A RESULT OF DIABETES AND AN ORGAN TRANSPLANT

1. primary care physician
2. nephrologist
3. endocrinologist
4. cardiologist
5. dermatologist
6. vascular specialist
7. podiatrist
8. ophthalmologist
9. retina specialist
10. orthopedic doctor (orthopedist)
11. endodontist (dental)
12. oral surgeon
13. urologist
14. alternative medicine / naturopathic physicians
15. massage therapist

I have asked God if He wants to "take me," let it be like my grandfather and grandmother (who were together for more than sixty years). On Thanksgiving Day after dinner my grandmother said, "I'm going to take a nap now," and she never woke up. And my grandfather, three years later because of the grief of missing his complement, lay down and went to "the other side" the same way. But, as always, if through my suffering someone else can be helped, then God's perfect will be done.

June 21, 2012

What Went Wrong With A Kidney Transplant On January 13, 2011

This is one of the bad things that can happen in organ transplant to the donor. This actually happened on January 13, 2011. Surgeons in University Medical Center in Lubbock, Texas used dysfunctional clips on Florinda Gotcher, a 41-year-old mother of four, who gave one of her kidneys to her brother. The clip broke off from an artery, and she died about 30 minutes after surgery. This death could have been avoided.

A CNN.com article by John Bonifield and Elizabeth Cohen of CNN, posted on June 21, 2012, stated:

> Starting in 2004, transplant surgeons, such as Dr. Amy Friedman, began raising concerns about using clips in kidney donors, sending letters to the U.S. Food and Drug Administration and making presentations at transplant conferences and publishing articles in medical journals.

According to the article, since 2001 four others have died from these malfunctioning clips and twelve were seriously injured. You may want to check to see who the manufacturer was, because they could have put stronger warnings on the boxes and the packages, as there are none! The warning is one line in multiple pages of instructions, in a separate package, with a different surgical tool that is used for putting the clips on.

The F.D.A. knew about these deaths since 2001 and said they sent warning letters to hospitals and to this particular hospital. But evidently something went wrong with the four others who have died and the twelve who were injured. As I said previously in this book, in the bureaucracy of the medical field, the right hand often does not know what the left hand is doing.

So you might want to <u>ask questions</u>. Some hospitals may be still using the clips because the left hand, again, does not know what the right hand is doing, and the letters of warning might go unheeded.

We pray for her brother, whom I am sure is in terrible grief. If this would have happened to my daughter, I do not think that I would want to live. So I am sure this terrible tragedy affected her whole family for the rest of their lives—especially her sister who is on the video and, of course, her four children.

For more information, see the article titled "Kidney-Donor Deaths Linked To Surgical Clips Raise Issues Of Alerts, Warnings" and video on cnn.com at:

http://cnn.com/2012/06/20/health/kidney-clips/ index.html?hpt=hp_c1 (center)

If they take the video off CNN.com, you may check for it on YouTube.

September 27, 2012

I went to my nephrologist today, Dr. Joy Logan, and she gave me some scary news. It seems that I have a BK virus, something that doctors have realized in the last ten years most people have. But with 25% of Dr. Logan's kidney transplant patients this virus is more deadly because it attacks the new kidney due to their natural immune system being suppressed by the immunosuppressants that I and other kidney transplant patients are taking to keep the body from rejecting our new kidneys.

She conferred with Dr. Kaplan of the University of Arizona Kidney Transplant Team. To keep from losing my kidney, we chose a method to reduce the immunosuppressants to two pills per day (I'm taking mycophenolate 250 mg. now), so that my natural immune system can keep the BK virus at bay. This of course can result in losing my kidney anyway.

The doctor has to add the steroid Prednisone to my other immunosuppressant drugs, and this will cause me to be more hungry and grumpy (the immunosuppressants are already causing grumpiness) and crave sweets, which can cause high sugars that will also attack my organs and my new kidney. This may not be so for others.

While this would all seem pretty devastating to the average person who just received a kidney transplant, I must confess even myself, being a man of faith, I have to constantly remember who my God is. My first question was "Why even give people kidney transplants if this BK virus pops up to attack

25% of the patients?" At this point I have to do more research myself before I can write much more.

Perhaps this is God's way of allowing this BK virus to activate in my body so that I can get off of the immunosuppressants, because they're also causing osteoporosis in my bones. So I guess at this point I feel like a cosmic guinea pig. Is God allowing these things to happen to me so that I can write about it? I have to go in twice a month now for blood tests, so I definitely can't get away from those needles.

I asked how soon a person would know if he was going into renal failure, and the doctor said that they can't always tell right away and that usually the blood tests detect it. What I didn't find out for sure (and she didn't offer the information) is if it's possible to go into renal failure right away, suddenly, and die before they can get me to a dialysis center. Truthfully, I've thought through this one too, and as I said at the end of (the first edition) of the book, I probably would want to die rather than go back to the dialysis. So God—knowing all of this—has to continue working a miracle in my life, if He wants me on this side serving humanity.

October 19, 2012

On October 18, 2012 the blood tests came back which says my kidney is still functioning normally. So far so good. However, I am gaining much weight because the steroid medicine, called Prednisone, makes me always hungry.

November 12, 2012

On October 23, 2012 I went in for blood tests again. On November 7, 2012 I saw my nephrologist Dr. Logan, and she shared that the BK virus was down to normal. She is recommending, through Dr. Kaplan at the university hospital, to reduce my Prednisone, which acts like an immunosuppressant but eats away at my bone marrow.

I also have been very very tired as of late. Today I have started this reduction. We shall see what happens. I won't be seeing Dr. Logan again until the beginning of the new year.

November 27, 2012

On November 27, 2012 the blood draws were still normal.

December 18, 2012

On December 18, 2012 the blood draws were still normal.

January 18, 2013

Visit with Dr. Logan: She said that my kidney was still 70% healthy, which was very high. However the Prednisone was still causing bone deterioration, which is why I felt my legs getting weaker. She wanted me to go back for blood tests the next week, which I did.

January 25, 2013

Blood tests: About a week later, Dr. Logan called and said that my sugars were off the charts and needed to drastically come down. So my insulin was increased in order to save the kidney from damage from high sugars. I also have to watch what my carbohydrate intake is.

Now I have the fear that my pancreas is failing. I already know that my insurance will not pay for that operation, or my heart possibly not be able to withstand that operation.

June 14, 2013

Dr. Andrew Weil, in his own way—without completely leaving the system—is making some alternative inroads in the medical field, and he is right here in Tucson, Arizona. I hope you take the time to get the 2012 film *Escape Fire: The Fight to Rescue American Healthcare*, to see what he is up to. It will be worth the watching, particularly for young doctors and health practitioners who are looking for alternative methods of healing as well as organizations to work for, or even to start their own healing institute, like I did in starting the Soulistic Medical Institute and Hospice.

Which reminds me, the heavily increasing burden of Federal and State regulations and financial penalties for infractions is making it increasingly difficult for small hospices to survive, as the large hospices have employees to meet these regulations and financial means that the small hospices do not have. This puts a lot of unnecessary pressure on all the dedicated workers who are willing to work for less money and fewer benefits in order to work for a small hospice, so they can give more individualized care to the patients. For sure, these big hospice corporations had somebody write something into law to try to drive out small hospices. If you are in a position of governmental authority that can help change this law, please accept this responsibility, before God, to do so. Please contact your Senator or Congressman.

July 12, 2013

With diabetes, for most unfortunate people who have it, it is a slow death. One thing goes, and then another organ or eye, or a heart problem pops up. It is definitely faith over fear. It is a long teaching, and this is not the book for that. This week I saw a cardiologist, and he tells me there is tissue on one of the muscles on my heart—an enlarged heart muscle. The medical term is dyspnea. But I have a new pill to try to help deal with that.

Yet I know that ultimately it is my mind over my body and my faith in God over the pills that I take, whatever those pills are. I am not adverse, of course, to any prescribed medications. I do think, however, that a lot of them are unnecessary, and the pharmaceutical companies make a lot of money on unnecessary drugs that they want doctors to prescribe to patients. So I ask a lot of questions.

This week also I saw the eye doctor, who had to again do laser surgery on my good eye—not because it is bleeding now, but because I have water on the eye due to diabetic macular degeneration. I have little fears here and there about losing my good eye, but that is just, again, the battle between faith over fear. Many people succumb to the fear, and then the body manifests the disease a lot faster. I know I am in God's hands. I am of course trying to watch my eating of the wrong foods.

The good news is, with my continued blood tests, my kidney is still functioning almost 100% after two years now since the transplant. I do suggest people read my book *Teachings On Healing, From A Spiritual Perspective*, written by Niánn Emerson Chase and me. I am sixty-seven years old, and I am still performing with my eleven-piece Bright & Morning Star Band. I cannot stand up any more while performing because of the neuropathy, and I cannot hit those high notes, but I can still sing in my unique style and do a complete two-hour concert. James Gandolfini recently died at age fifty-one of an apparent heart attack, according to the news, but I believe he also had diabetes. So I am doing pretty good, still being alive, functioning in my mind as an administrator and musician at sixty-seven.

September 4, 2013

Between the last writing and this one, I found out that I had a cataract in my good eye, which has caused the blurriness that I have been experiencing for the last several months. You would think that the retina specialist would have seen this. But, no, he was not looking for cataracts on the surface. The only reason I found out is I went to get new eyeglasses and had an eye examination with the optometrist who detected the cataract. So I had the cataract removed, and low and behold the blurriness is gone and I can see better now!

My nephrologist thinks that I should go back and get another tube put down my throat to look for possible damaged ducts in my stomach. Now you would think they would have looked the last time they went down my throat. But, no, that would be the common sense thing to do—to look for anything that might be wrong, once they invade a person's throat and stomach.

June 2, 2014

I continue to see my nephrologist, Dr. Logan, and all seems to be well, particularly not getting again the BK virus. My weight continues to stay at about 198-199 lbs., which I feel is way too much for my little 5'5" body. I still feel it's because of the immunosuppressant drugs I'm taking and the inflamed stomach I have all the time, although I've been really trying to eat the right things. Being raised to eat all the wrong things, it is very difficult to break these habits in your older years. So when you take immunosuppressants, you really do have to stay off the carbohydrates, sugars, and heavy meats (which are hard to digest).

And with the added problem of neuropathy and my limping problem (due to the Cottonwood, Arizona orthopedic doctor causing my leg to be shortened in the surgical repairing of a fractured hip), I can hardly stand on my feet now and can walk very little without my legs feeling like they want to cave in. That surgeon never did respond to my requests to make any effort to repair my short leg now.

My wife, TiyiEndea, is having her own orthopedic nightmares with her doctor in Tucson, who—the last time she went to him—was actually rude to her, as well as his assistant, saying TiyiEndea's problem was not even with her hip; it's with her back. He did replace her one hip and knows that her other hip is bad, due to her being a gymnast when she was younger, which caused damage.

In the past, this doctor gave her two steroid shots to relieve the pain and now is saying he doesn't want to give her anymore, because it will affect her new hip, if and when he ever decides to give her one. Basically he's telling her to live with the pain now and even denying it is her other hip. If anyone knows her body, it is TiyiEndea, who is a midwife and very in tune with her body. He told her she should just walk with a cane. Excuse me? She's only 50, and looks 40! She did write him and expressed her feelings, and he did call her back and agreed to give her another steroid shot to help ease her pain.

Anyway, orthopedic doctors really stick with one another. I went to TiyiEndea's doctor myself in the past, to see if he could do anything with my short leg, and—like another doctor before TiyiEndea's (who was also an orthopedic doctor)—he said, "Well, your Cottonwood doctor could have done something else, but what he did was OK." I said,

"How could it be OK if I am walking with a limp now?"

The point is that they cover each other's behinds, because they are so afraid of being sued. In those cases they are not trying to do what is best for the patient; they are trying to lessen the possibilities of a lawsuit. It is almost impossible to prove that a doctor indeed made a mistake because there are very few colleagues, or expert witnesses, who would testify to the fault of the doctor. They all seem to have the same rote answer. On the streets it's called "bullshit."

My advice when dealing with all orthopedic doctors is the boxing rule: "to protect yourself at all times" and do as much research as you can before you get a fracture fixed, or a hip replacement, or knee surgery, or anything. And if you have a broken hip and are rushed to Emergency and if you are passed out, have your loved one ask "is this operation going to shorten my loved one's leg or cause other negative side effects?" And if they say yes, ask if there is another way.

In closing

There is much research being done for a cure for cancer and many other diseases. I hope that there will be more research done for repairing nerves that have been destroyed by neuropathy. Of course I think prevention is much better than tackling any disease once it has taken root in the body. This is why I wrote this book, to hopefully prevent people from getting diabetes and all its complications. What is really needed is nutritional education and a change in the consciousness of Americans, who eat foods full of toxins, including GMOs (Genetically Modified Organisms), which not enough is known about. Americans need to get back to home gardens, grown without poisonous fertilizers and pesticides.

    We, as a nation, need to be leaders in the world in sustainability in our eating and energy-saving. There is much information available now about our decaying and unsustainable planetary environment. The body is a vehicle that needs pure energy, and when it is fed toxins, it malfunctions—so does the mind, and so does the soul. Everything is related, as many indigenous tribes know. You might not be able to change the whole world by yourself, but you can change yourself and what you teach your children.

PART 2

THE HIGH COST OF HEALTHCARE: FROM BABIES TO HOSPICE

The following articles are reprinted from the Spring 2008 issue (Volume VI, Number 1) of the *Alternative Voice*, the theme of which focuses on "The High Cost of Healthcare: from Babies to Hospice."

The *Alternative Voice* is a quarterly publication that believes in creating global change by offering beginning solutions and addressing the many crises our world faces today—social, environmental, political, and spiritual. You can subscribe via:

Alternative Voice
P.O. Box 4910
Tubac, AZ 85646
(520) 603-9932

info@alternativevoice.org

alternativevoice.org

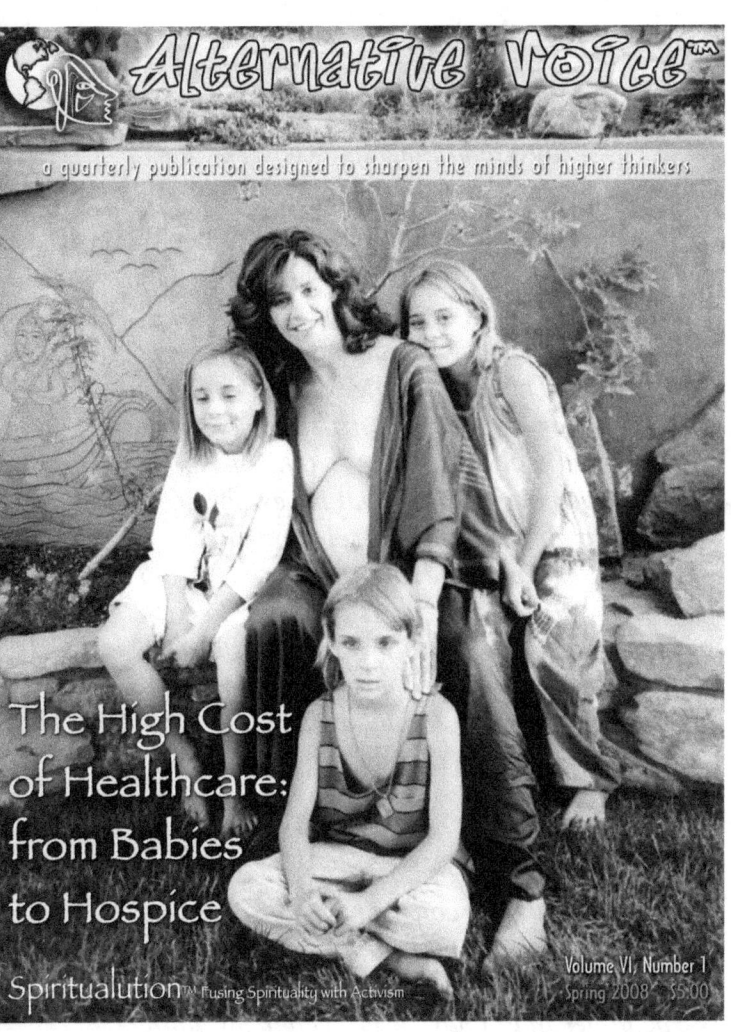

My wife TiyiEndea, my twin daughters SanSkritA & DeleVan, my son Amadon, and my daughter Ellanora DesManae in the womb, 1997

Eco-Systems, Social-Systems, And Person-Systems

by Niánn Emerson Chase

Recently I explained to my primary healthcare physician how I saw our relationship:

> *You are my physician, my only doctor at this time. This is my choice. I trust you over any other doctor when it comes to my personal health, but I also "tune in" to my own body and what I intuit is best for me. I see our doctor-patient relationship as a collaboration, a team effort, for it is not really up to you to solve my health problems, but up to me. You're there to assist me, and I value your experience, your knowledge, your wisdom, and your godliness. I know that you have my highest good in mind when you act as my physician, and I trust you. I won't always agree with your opinions or suggestions, but I will always consider them.*
>
> *In spite of my physical aging process and increased limitations, I think I am healthier than I have ever been in my entire life. My overall health just keeps getting better because my psychospiritual health just keeps getting better. I feel strong and more balanced physically, emotionally, intellectually, and spiritually than ever before. Though I no longer can do certain*

things physically that I could do fifteen or twenty years ago, I can do many other things that I couldn't do two decades ago, mostly on the intellectual and psychospiritual levels.

You are my dear beloved physician, friend, and fellow minister. You have been an integral part of my ongoing improving overall health and well-being. Thank you, my doctor friend, for your dedicated love, humility, flexibility, openness, and collaboration in this continuing process of remaining healthy. I feel blessed by God to have you by my side in a physician's role, and I hope that all of your other patients have similar sentiments.

I realize that most patients don't feel that way about their doctors, at least in this country. But there have always been some exceptional doctors in every generation, doctors who are in the ministry of caring for the well-being of others rather than in the business of healthcare. My primary-care doctor, Dr. Landau Lawrence, is one of those exceptional people, and so are others from the past as well as in the present. These exceptional ones are of various races, religions, and nationalities and include both men and women.

Many physicians, psychologists, nurses, and patients have something to say about the state of the healthcare system in this country, based on their own personal experiences and thoroughly researched facts. Some go a step further and realize that healthcare should involve an integration of considering the whole person, which includes the entire physical body-system, as well as the emotional-, mental-, and spirit-systems of the individual.

Interestingly, as an avid student and teacher of the concepts found in *The URANTIA Book*, I have noted that when referring to the health of a person, this wonderful spiritually-based text associates "health" with the body, mind, and soul. Health is linked with sensible living habits, happiness, mental clarity, emotional stability, and an awareness of spiritual reality.

> *Health, sanity [mental efficiency], and happiness are integrations of truth, beauty, and goodness as they are blended in human experience. Such levels of efficient [balanced] living come about through the unification of the energy [physical] systems, idea [mind] systems, and spirit systems.*[1]

Rather than compartmentalizing human beings into separate parts to be "treated" by specialists, exceptional healthcare givers/ministers have more of a "wholistic" perspective when interacting with those they are attempting to aid in becoming healthier by integrating and unifying and blending parts rather than separating them out.

The more progressive healthcare providers, scientists, sociologists, educators, theologians, and statespersons (rather than mere politicians) realize that in treating "sick" environments, societies, and persons you have to look at the entire eco-systems, social-systems, and person-systems. The declining health of Mother Earth matches and is interlinked with the declining health of our modern societies and individual citizens.

In my own struggles to maintain good health and well-being, I have discovered that my own life-support systems seem to match the Earth's and its peoples. As the lungs of the Earth are being debilitated by the massive destruction of rain forests, my lungs feel compromised too. As the Earth's waterways are being poisoned and depleted, so does my circulatory system feel sluggish and inefficient. As people's hearts are broken and their spirits diminished by a consumer-driven, mechanistic social system, so my heart feels fragile with my grieving over the cold-hearted state of the dominant culture.

I think that poor health—whether in a person or in our natural world or in a society—is a result of being out of divine pattern. Divine pattern involves integrative systems that all coordinate to reflect the truth, beauty, and goodness of God, and, frankly, a vast majority of religious endeavors and institutions on this world are not healthy at all, regardless of their religious rhetoric. They are very sick and have been out of divine pattern for many thousands of years.

Tens of thousands of years ago the ancient Sethite priesthood was comprised of "high-minded and noble teachers of health and religion" who were "true educators" and not at all like most of the "debased" and "commercialized" religious teachers and healthcare providers of today.[2] Socrates and his successors, Plato and Aristotle, taught that goodness was the *health of the soul*.[3] Today, only a few healthcare professionals—who are caught in the ocean of a grasping, greedy medical industrial complex—realize the truth that people's health is tied up with the state of their souls.

The work that I am involved in, which encompasses every aspect of my life, integrates all life experiences into a whole. My own healing process has been one of becoming uncompartmentalized and more unified within my whole being. The Soulistic Medical Institute, which is a facet of my work, has another way of looking at "health." It has redefined health in its outreach ministries of providing healthcare, just as I have had to continually redefine what good health is for me as I unfold into my God-given personality circuitry and grow psychospiritually.

In my own health-maintenance process I rarely use "health professionals" and medicines because I don't need to. Though very full with meaningful work and many responsibilities, my lifestyle is less strenuous and rushed than twenty years ago. I eat organically-grown foods from our Avalon Gardens; drink clean, chemical-free water from our private wells; exercise by daily walking and hiking in beautiful natural places; and use eco-friendly common products for home, lawn, and personal care. In not using toxic "foods" and products, I don't poison myself or my natural environment. And I feel good mentally in taking responsibility for caring for my physical health and for my natural environment.

Even more importantly, in taking responsibility for my own health is the overseeing of my psychospiritual welfare. I spend time reading and expanding intellectually. I interact closely with fellow kindred spirits and good friends in an intentional-community setting. And I laugh—at myself and at the many silly situations in life on this world.

Dr. Patch Adams is renown for his use of humor in the treatment of diseases and health promotion, as are certain teachers of spiritual truths. *The URANTIA Book* states: "Humor serves a valuable purpose both as a health insurance and as a liberator of emotional pressure, thus preventing injurious nervous tension and overserious contemplation."[4]

In the maintenance of my own health, I rest, contemplate, meditate, reflect, pray, and worship. I have come to fully embrace the truth that an understanding at some level of spiritual reality can contribute to the enjoyment of abundant health and to the cure of numerous mental, emotional, and nervous ailments.

Even the physical problems of bodily health and efficiency are best solved when they are viewed from the religious standpoint of our Master's [Jesus'] teaching: That the body and mind of mortals are the dwelling place of the gift of the Gods, the Spirit of God becoming the spirit of man and woman. The mind of men and women becomes the mediator between material

> *things and spiritual realities.*[5]
>
> *The joy of the outpoured spirit, when it is consciously experienced in human life, is a tonic for health, a stimulus for mind, and an unfailing energy for the soul.*[6]

Cellular biologist Dr. Bruce Lipton emphasizes that our beliefs can change how our genes will respond. He states: "The new science has everything to do with your beliefs." Though Dr. Lipton calls this awareness "new science," the fact that energy follows thought has been known in the circles of genuine religious persons for thousands of years.

Now with the new science a small number of progressive scientists and healthcare professionals are beginning to understand the power of thought and how energy in body systems is affected by the state of mind in individuals. With thinking and attitudes that are founded on truth, beauty, and goodness, there is a greater probability for healing. Beliefs and perspectives that are negative, resentful, self-centered, and fear-based can cause poor health. In addition, the beliefs and energy fields of other people around an individual can affect how healthy or unhealthy that individual will be.

If our perceptions determine the status of our well-being, if our thoughts as well as the thoughts of those around us can create disease or healing, wouldn't we want to be extremely aware of what healthcare providers we allow into our lives? Wouldn't we want to be more selective of the places we go to when we are sick and who we hang out with when we are trying to get better? Wouldn't we want to become more educated about what goes on behind the scenes in the medical industrial complex? Wouldn't we want to know what the mindset *really* is within the American Medical Association, the huge pharmaceutical corporations, the Federal Drug Administration (FDA), the medical insurance companies, and most hospitals?

Read on, to not only identify the problem but to gain a vision of a wholer and healthier life.

Niánn Emerson Chase (descendant of Ralph Waldo Emerson) is a co-founder of Global Community Communications Alliance as well as the Soulistic Medical Institute in Tubac, Arizona and Soulistic Hospice in Tubac and Tucson, Arizona.

The Truth and Answers About Free Healthcare

by Gabriel of Urantia

Jesus wasn't a politician. However, I recently [Spring 2008] watched both Democratic and Republican debates. I was hoping to watch a third-party debate, but that's another article. Maybe ten minutes of the more than four hours of presentations were spent on the need for free national healthcare. And in those ten minutes, from all of the candidates, I think I understood about 5 seconds of their 26-letter, bureaucratic jargon—jargon that really means nothing. As the Native American elders would say, "They speak with forked tongue."

In order to talk about "free" anything, you have to realize what the root of the problem is. And that is: plain greed. You see, doctors are supposed to be healers. They are supposed to go into the profession because of a calling from God, not for the desire to become rich or to have top status in a broken and materialistic society.

I've known of or met few true doctors in my life. Albert Schweitzer was a true doctor. Patch Adams is a true doctor. The several doctors who recently treated my son for a serious health situation are true doctors. Dr. Landau Lawrence—with Soulistic Medical Institute in Tubac, Arizona—is a true doctor. Of course, there are others I haven't met or heard of. Dr. Landau still makes house calls! How many doctors still do that? If you ask that of "doctors" today, they will think you are kidding.

What a weird concept, for a doctor to come and visit the sick!

Many physicians get caught up in a system perpetuated by greed, due to: first, the schools they attend and the high cost of becoming a state-certified doctor, and then interning in hospitals that they then spend the rest of their lives associated with.

A large majority of the hospitals are privately owned and function under the capitalistic policy of profit. As a matter of fact, if you can't pay, you just might die. You may ask yourself this question: "Why would a doctor or a healthcare facility do that?" I guess we can also ask: "Why would a person with a scientific mind work for a government or corporation making nuclear bombs and other weapons of chemical and biological warfare?" So, perhaps privatization and public health should not be mentioned in the same breath.

I think that in a government that is truly "for the people, by the people, and of the people," in that kind of republic, democracy should take care of the health needs of its citizens. So what has happened?

As it is in the media and the entertainment business, so it is in health services—privatization and monopolization have become the rule. This happens over time because of the inequality of social status (which includes wages, education, and opportunity) as well as many other factors.

As I've said before, at the root of these evils are greed and the pursuit of power, which I would call *dio power*, as opposed to a good kind of power that I would call *Deo power* or God-given power to help others. In Western civilization, most schools perpetrate dio power from first grade to doctorate levels, and it manifests in every career because these institutions are so much a part of the larger society or system that is steeped in dio-power-oriented materialism.

Many altruistic students who graduate with a degree in social services and get a job in "the system" soon discover the inequality of the system. I know that I may be saying things that you've already heard and even experienced, but I'm trying to put it in relation to an answer to the problems.

You see, people have to change and have to stop supporting those in the system who perpetuate the lie. What really needs to change are the hearts of people.

The true "Great American Dream" had to do with freedom and concern for its citizenry, not for individual wealth at the expense of others. Somehow this dream got twisted to imply that individuals had the right to make as much money as they could (regardless of negative impacts on land and society), basically benefiting from slave labor. In this method, which is still dominant worldwide, the rich get richer and the poor get poorer.

We have to start thinking more on a planetary level. The "Great American Dream" needs to become the "Great Planetary Dream." We need to start seeing all people of all nations as our brothers and sisters, as stated in this phrase I have coined:

We are all one planetary family.

I think the answer in all of Western civilization, and indeed the world, is pretty simple: we need more standardized and fair salaries, straight across the board.

Who's more important: the architect or the carpenter? Without the carpenter's hands-on labor, you wouldn't have a house to live in. An idea is great, and putting it down on paper is a gift. But you also need the gifted carpenters to build it.

Who's more important: the sports hero (who gets to play games all his life, like many of us did before we had to grow up) or the teacher (who intellectually nourishes and hopefully inspires your children)? Why should the sports hero make millions of dollars per year and the teacher receive a barely-survivable income?

Who's more important: the owner of a supermarket chain or the farmer? Without the farmer, there would be no food in the supermarket.

Who's more important: the car designer or the mechanic (who fixes it when it breaks down)?

Who's more important: the rock star (who all too often becomes a star because of being willing to compromise his or her music and ideals and live a lifestyle of moral decadence) or the non-compromising musician (who is barely able to make a living because he or she won't stoop to those levels of compromise and immorality, who just wants to create beautiful music)?

Who's more important: the doctor of American-Medical-Association (A.M.A.) mentality (who supposedly diagnoses your illness and prescribes certain drugs to fix you—drugs you can't afford in the first place) or the true healer (who tries to get to the root of the problem and prescribes proper thinking, herbs, diet, exercise, and a holistic health program, which includes preventative measures)?

How many doctors have told you that you've got to change your attitude in order to heal? That you have to be a nicer person, a more giving person, or whatever they intuit about your dio (erroneous and selfish) thinking and behavior? As Ralph Waldo Emerson stated: "What lies before us and what lies behind us is not so important as what lies within us."

In many states certain alternative healing practices are considered illegal, and authors who write books about alternative healing methods have to protect themselves with statements like the one below from the book, *The Yeast Syndrome* by John P. Trowbridge and Morton Walker.

> *Be aware that nutritional dosages for food supplements which exceed the recommended dietary allowances of the National Research Council of the U. S. National Academy of Sciences represent a therapeutic intervention and should be taken only under the direction of a properly trained and experienced holistic physician.*

Accordingly, the coauthors and the publisher offer this disclaimer:

> *Information presented in this book is not to be construed as the practice of medicine or the giving of medical advice.*

We are not practicing nutritional therapy, which is illegal in certain states of the United States. . . .

If you watch the early evening news on any of the major networks, you are inundated with approximately fifteen minutes worth of commercials in a half-hour program. In those fifteen minutes you will see a "quick fix"—in pill form—advertised for every disease and discomfort known to modern man, and some that are made up. If there isn't something wrong with you, after seeing all of those commercials, you can't help but begin to think you need a pill.

One of my favorite made-up diseases is the "restless legs" syndrome. I've got a free answer to that one: instead of taking a pill full of synthetic materials that cause all kinds of side effects, simply get up and go for a walk! Get some exercise! Get that blood circulating! And you might want to look at your diet too!

The pharmaceutical companies—closely linked to the A.M.A.—make billions of dollars trying to convince you you're sick somewhere in your body. Their lobbyists and lawyers work very hard against any kind of alternative healthcare or common-sense, holistic healing.

Perhaps a way to help change the system is to find "true" doctors, "true" healers who aren't trying to get rich on you and your loved ones, and go to them for help with your health problems. Give your support to those healing practitioners (which do include some physicians) who are trying to make a living in a moderate manner while helping others heal and develop health-promoting lifestyles and habits.

How can you find a decent way to make a living without being caught up in greed and desires for an unsustainable lifestyle that not only causes poor health for you but for many others too?

Capitalism in itself is not wrong, but it's how it is used by those desiring too big of a piece of the world-resources pie. There's nothing the matter with using capital as a means of exchange. It's the value that some people put on their so-called talents that is way out of whack. How rich do you have to be? How about rich enough to support you and your family and live comfortably? The problem is what some people consider "comfortable". I guess that's going to have to be between you and God.

The problem is that there are many people who have no idea what God wants them to do or even care to know! You see, if you trust God and not mammon (material wealth), God will provide for you and your family. He will take care of all your needs, but not necessarily your wants. Now this doesn't mean that you don't have to do anything to support yourself and your family; it means that if your trust comes from Godly principles rather than principles based on greed and selfishness, you will find worthwhile work.

In the dio system, we are bombarded by corporate-controlled media to desire things we don't really need—things made and sold by those who advertise with the media. This has everything to do with healthcare because healthcare is part of a whole system that needs to change. This all-encompassing system, of which medical concerns are a part, needs to become a system in concern for other people, not just for ourselves.

Basically the answer is living the first two commandments which are:

Love the Lord your God with all your heart, mind, and soul. And then your neighbor as yourself.

Wow! What an idea! If this could be followed by doctors, governmental leaders, politicians, corporate executives, educators, professionals of all careers, laborers, and religious leaders, there would be free healthcare, free education, and a lot of other things free.

So, you're thinking, "This will never happen." But it can happen, beginning with you. Join those who have already applied this divine principle to their lives. There are people doing it. We need to find each other. We need to form communities outside of the system. We need to barter with each other. We need to be givers instead of takers. And we need to also realize the simple truth that I coined for our religious community to follow:

Your child is my child, and my child is yours.

You can take this truth another step:

Your grandmother and grandfather are my grandmother and grandfather, and your mother and father are my mother and father.

In this manner, we begin to care more for each other. Under this simple but profound thinking, we realize that "nationalism" breaks down to family, and we are all one planetary family under God. With that kind of thinking, worldwide cooperation, peace, and harmony will eventually evolve.

This is not an impossible dream; this is the future. This is the new millennium that is coming, which *The URANTIA Book* calls the first stage of light and life.

Evil will work itself out within people, because people will begin to see that it doesn't work. It doesn't work in their own lives, and it doesn't work for the good of humanity. People will begin to make right and higher choices. It is happening now. And it is happening at an accelerated rate.

Maybe you're one of those unhappy doctors or dentists who would rather be a coach or a cook or an athlete or an actor, or whatever, but you're trapped with bills and kids to support. Or you want to be a doctor, but you can't really heal anyone because you're trapped in the system of formulas for prescribed medicines, many in which you really don't believe can bring a cure or healing.

Here's a phenomenal idea: QUIT! It's better to have bad credit or no credit at all for a while than to develop a bad heart or the manifestation of another disease.

Trust your higher dreams. And most of all trust God, the Originator of idealistic dreams that, when realized, would contribute to your and others' good health—physically, mentally, and spiritually. With faith and trust in God and in making choices that are for the good of others, God will help you fulfill those dreams of altruism and morality. But you must begin to take the first baby steps of faith, away from a system that doesn't work—for you, your children, or humanity.

Gabriel of Urantia is co-founder of Global Community Communications Alliance as well as the Soulistic Medical Institute in Tubac, Arizona and Soulistic Hospice in Tubac and Tucson, Arizona.

The Medical Industrial Complex
*by Marayeh Cunningham, Ph.D.,
Clinical Psychologist*

The *ministry of healing* has been transformed into the "medical industrial complex" (as Dr. Brent James calls it). It has become one of the most profitable businesses on the planet rather than remaining a healing ministry and profession. With false promises and deceptive advertising, the medical industrial complex preys on people's desire to be truly healed and/or to have their loved ones healed.

Corporate greed has swallowed healthcare. Large corporations have gobbled up what were once a wide variety of small businesses in every area of healthcare including the pharmaceutical industry, medical insurance industry, hospitals, medical laboratories, and imaging centers. Physicians are no longer in charge of healthcare, as they were until recently. Today the gigantic healthcare industry has taken over, emphasizing profit rather than health. The reality is that the corporations are now in charge of our healthcare, and their reason "to be" is for creating profit, not to promote health.

Today, people often blindly trust the doctors. Doctors, in turn, rely on the drug reps. The drug reps, plain and simple, are just SALESMEN! They don't have any license or medical training. They just are good at selling a product, and pharmaceuticals today are being marketed just like any other product—such as cars or perfume—where a desire for the product is created and the manufacturers of these products deliberately and consciously exaggerate their benefits and minimize their drawbacks (just like all manufacturers and sellers of products do).

Pharmaceutical companies (Big Pharma) are in the business of making a profit. The more product they sell, and at the highest possible price, the more money they make, and pharmaceutical companies are some of the most profitable companies on the planet!

Commercialization

With this corporate takeover, the ethical foundations of medicine are severely endangered. The soul of the profession is eroding and being replaced by the profit motive. A major reason for this is the growing commercialization of the U.S. healthcare system:

- Healthcare has become a $2.2 trillion industry, largely shaped by corporations with profit rather than the interest of the patient as their main goal. In no other healthcare system in the world does the profit motive play such an important role. This is destabilizing the entire economy and eroding the ethical commitments of physicians.
- The United States now spends more on healthcare than it does on food.
- Despite higher costs, the United States does not deliver objectively better quality and

access for U.S. citizens relative to peer countries.

- The pharmaceutical industry has profits of more than three times that of the average of other Fortune 500 companies, even after including all research and development costs.
- Until 1980, the American Medical Association had held that "the practice of medicine should not be commercialized, nor treated as a commodity in trade." These sentiments reflecting the spirit of professionalism are now gone.
- Another commercializing force has been the growing influence of the pharmaceutical industry on the practice of medicine. This industry now uses its enormous financial resources to help shape the postgraduate and continuing medical education of physicians in ways that serve its marketing purposes. A medical profession that is being educated by an industry that sells the drugs physicians prescribe and other tools physicians use is abdicating its ethical commitment to serve as the independent guardian for its patients.
- The salaries of the healthcare corporations' CEOs are huge, with six- and seven-figure "bonuses" to the CEOs of major healthcare corporations.
- Insurance companies with record profits deny coverage to patients.

- Pharmaceutical companies, with some of the highest profit returns and with advertising budgets the size of third world countries' Gross Domestic Product, are pricing their drugs so high that many people cannot afford them.

The Insurance Industry

Our current medical insurance industry is very wasteful and expensive to the patient but very profitable to the insurance industry. Universal/single-payer coverage challenges corporate-dominated healthcare. With universal coverage, access to healthcare is a right for all people. Such a system alters the profit motives alive in the corporate for-profit system that is now in place. That is why there is so much opposition to it.

The profit motive has become totally dominate over the delivery and quality of healthcare; it is what drives the medical industrial complex. Physicians are paid by the procedure not by the results. Corporations are legally obligated to protect investors' interests.

- With the present U.S. healthcare insurance, there is little incentive for the insurance companies to practice preventative medicine, as most with insurance stay with a given insurance company for less than six years.
- The United States is the richest country in the world and has a population of 300

million, and yet nearly 48 million Americans have no health insurance.
- Studies estimate that the number of excess deaths among uninsured adults age 25-64 is in the range of 18,000 a year.
- Insured patients are increasingly facing bigger deductibles. In 2005 the average annual deductible for a singe person employed by a small firm was $929.
- Doctors in the U.S. pay an estimated average of $27,500 a year for malpractice insurance.
- We spend $6,800 per American per year on healthcare. This is 16% of our gross domestic product (GDP), and it is rapidly increasing.
- A typical family of four spends almost as much on the health insurance premium as they do on their mortgage payment on the median American home, a $210,000 home. That's roughly twice of what the rest of the world spends.

Skyrocketing High Costs

Why are health costs so high in the United States?

- **The Profit Motive** – The private component of the U.S. healthcare system results in a $75 billion profit. Large pharmaceutical companies, technology companies, and medical laboratories develop a new product that they argue will improve someone's health, when in fact the real motive is profit. The problem is that very often the amount of benefit is tiny and the cost is huge. Sometimes the side effects are also very harmful. Big Pharma invests huge amounts of money in political campaigns, lobbying, and media campaigns to keep the profitable system "as is," and they are very invested in not seeing it change in such a way as to reduce their profits.

- **Lack of Rationing Care** – Almost half of healthcare spending is used to treat just 5% of the population. Much of this is spent in the last 6 months of life with futile attempts to save dying patients at astronomical costs. In the United States, people, not care, are rationed.
- **Bureaucracy** – The bureaucracy of the U.S. system incurs additional multiple-state and multiple-payer administrative structures. The extreme complexity of the different health plans is overwhelming, with constantly changing rules.

From a business point of view, healthcare is very successful, growing much more rapidly than the GDP, but as a ministry to people it is a dismal failure. It is hard to put a figure on the cost of the mental anguish caused by the financial burden placed on people and the stress of not getting effective care because people can't afford it.

- Healthcare debt is responsible for half of the bankruptcies in the United States.
- The median U.S. family income is $48,999 a year, and some families are paying $12,000 a year for health insurance.
- Top-selling drugs of the leading pharmaceutical companies are on average 2.3 times more expensive in the U.S. than in other countries.

Pharmaceuticals And The FDA, Bedfellows

Of course, there are drugs that can be lifesaving or extremely beneficial, but increasingly the pharmaceutical companies are putting more and more drugs on the market just to make a huge profit, and some of these drugs are less effective and/or more harmful than existing drugs. They also often make decisions to not put the effort into developing drugs that could save millions of lives because they would not be profitable, such as anti-parasitic drugs to fight parasites that ravage some third-world countries.

Instead they concentrate on drugs that they market for people to take chronically and often for the rest of their life. Pharmaceutical companies spend millions and millions of dollars to promote/advertise drugs, and then when they go off patent (and thus become a generic drug), suddenly the promotion stops. In the wake of new drug after new drug entering the market place, we now find ourselves in an ocean of pills, wondering which one to take and why.

Drugs that have been on the market for years are much safer on average than newly-released and highly-advertised drugs, because drugs that have been on the market for years have been given time to see what the long-term effects may be. Also, after a drug has been on the market for many years, it goes off patent and becomes generic and is available at a more reasonable price.

Drug trials/testing often last for only 8-10 weeks. Yet these same shortly-tested drugs are then prescribed for long-term use to patients while no one has any idea of the long-term affects! The latest move to prescribe drugs designed for adults to children as young as two is alarming, especially for the psychotropic drugs where we have no information on how these drugs will affect the young developing brain over a lifetime.

- The Federal Drug Administration (FDA) does NOT conduct the clinical trials that are needed to test the safety and efficacy of a new drug in order to being it to market. The pharmaceutical company that wants to manufacture and market the drug does the studies to prove the safety and efficacy of the drug.

- Contradictory studies showing the drug does not work or has serious side effects are usually not published.

- Continuing medical education (CME) is required by state law for all doctors who must take a given number of hours of CME each year, and 80% or more of these courses

are funded by the drug industry and offered at no cost to the physician. So in reality, CME has become another extension of the marketing for the drug industry.
- Conflicts of interest are common on the Federal Drug Administration (FDA) committees that decide whether or not a drug can go on the market. All too often members on these committees hold stock in the manufacturing company for the drug or are paid consultants for the pharmaceutical company.

People look to physicians, government, the FDA, and our media for guidance with their health, and all of these point to the drug solution for health problems because of the influence of the drug industry—Big Pharma. So what we don't have is a real understanding of what are the most effective interventions and preventions for these diseases or conditions. These are important societal questions that we have handed over to the drug industry to answer with a simple "take a pill."

- In any given week four out of every five U.S. adults will use prescription medicines, over-the-counter drugs, or dietary supplements, and nearly one third of adults will take five or more different medications.
- The reason a license is needed to prescribe prescription medications is that these drugs can have serious negative side effects, and

your doctor is expected to weigh the advantages and disadvantages of you taking the drug.
- Few physicians have the time or training in research methodology and statistics to investigate the studies of the drugs they prescribe and instead rely on the drug reps, journal articles, CME lectures, and pharmaceutical advertising in medical journals.

I think that all clinical trials should be conducted by a firm that has no relationship whatsoever with the FDA or any pharmaceutical company. In fact, the testing firms' identity should be kept secret from the FDA and the pharmaceutical companies, the researchers should be paid so well, and the penalties for any influence from the FDA or pharmaceutical companies should be so great that there would be little temptation to bias the data.

- Merck & Co. will pay $4.85 billion into a fund to settle claims that Vioxx was responsible for causing myocardial infarction and stroke in patients who took the drug for pain. The settlement is for 50,000 claims because these patients suffered myocardial infarction or stroke within 14 days of taking the drug.
- Big Pharma fought against restrictions on direct-to-consumer advertising that has led to increased demand for drugs where drugs really shouldn't have been used, Vioxx being a classic example.

- Pharmaceutical companies often sponsor nonprofit groups to raise a cry about the terrible ravages of a particular disease, telling people about the symptoms of the disease and asking them to ask their doctor if something can be done about this. Then the doctor, who has been primed in order to prescribe the drug, may be saying *the patient is asking for it; I have to give them something*, and they write the prescription.
- There are physicians—who are paid by the pharmaceutical industry as speakers or who are doing research for the pharmaceutical industry and being paid by them as consultants—who sit on clinical practice guidelines committees determining how we should treat a certain disease. Then those clinical practice guidelines are printed in the most prestigious journals in their fields and are widely distributed by the drug representatives to individual practicing physicians all over the country.
- Many medical professional society's journals are being underwritten by advertising by the drug company. In some journals half of the journal is devoted to expensive pharmaceutical advertising. The articles in the journals often tout the benefits of these drugs. Many of these journals are sent to physicians free of charge, and it is the advertisers who pay for them.
- People who are in large part funded by the pharmaceutical industry and promoted by

the pharmaceutical industry end up becoming the key opinion leaders in their fields, and then end up writing the guidelines that other physicians read about in their professional journals and are expected to follow. It becomes a closed circle of information that is really influenced by the product manufacturers at every turn.

- As an example, if you look at the latest guidelines for obsessive compulsive disorder and how to treat this, ten out of the eleven physicians on the panel had conflicts of interest in that they had taken money from antidepressant manufacturers that had drugs for treating obsessive compulsive disorder.

The FDA has been remiss in their oversight and approval of drugs, largely as a result of under funding. There is a lack of assessment and evaluation of the person's total quality of life in the research. The side effects of these medications often negatively affect a person's quality of life and health, even though there may be some lifting of symptoms, or the person may not die from the disease the drug is treating but rather die from the side effects of the drug. Many medications have been over-hyped and over-marketed, due to greed in the pharmaceutical industry.

The FDA has allowed this by not insisting on much higher standards in research design and control of variables that obviously bias almost all of this research in favor of the pharmaceutical companies. The FDA's drug division gets nearly half of its revenue from the drug industry itself in the form of user fees earmarking the money be spent to speed up the approval of new drugs, but not allowing any of that money to be spent on oversight or follow up monitoring.

If the pharmaceutical companies are giving so much money to the FDA, can the FDA do its job properly? Is the FDA regulating the pharmaceutical industry or partnering with it?

Little long-term research has been done on most of these drugs before they go on the market. I think that drugs should not be widely marketed for prescribing for periods longer than they have clinical trials and follow-up research data for, or in age groups or with people with serious medical conditions whose reactions to these drugs have not been adequately tested. It is wrong to put drugs on the market after clinical trials of only four, six, or eight weeks when these drugs are almost always used considerably longer than that. There are potential long-term harmful effects that do not show up in one- and two-month trials. What will young children, whose brains and neural patterns are being formed, be like at forty? The answer is that we do not know. The FDA has been too influenced by the pharmaceutical industry to adequately protect the millions of people taking these drugs.

The FDA is greatly influenced by the pharmaceutical corporations, and they often allow drugs on the market that do more harm than good. The quality of the research designs is often poor; the population samples are in no way random but are highly screened rather than being a representative cross section of people likely to take the drug, and the drug companies do the research that is used to decide the efficacy and safety of these drugs.

Most physicians are unaware of the research used to approve these drugs and are very significantly effected by the extensive marketing to them. Few physicians are sufficiently trained in research methodology to understand the biased, and in some cases apparently unethical, methods in the research procedures used to approve drugs that have a high potential for harm. The physicians trust the FDA too much, and in turn, the patients trust the physicians too much, and thus they are not sufficiently aware of the dangers and minimal benefits of many of the drugs that are being prescribed for them.

The Medicalised Society

Our society is largely encouraged by the current healthcare system to rely on Big Pharma's "solutions" for any conditions that may arise.

- A large percentage of chronic disorders are the normal consequences of poor habits or poor childrearing practices that need to be corrected with education and people taking responsibility for their lives. These are not diseases that require prescription medications but lifestyle changes. They require EFFORT and isn't it so much easier, for everyone involved, to just take a pill?!

- About 10% of school-age children are diagnosed with Attention Deficit/Hyperactivity Disorder (ADHA) and treated with dugs that have toxic side effects. The production of drugs to treat ADHA has risen 2,000% in nine years!
- Psychotropic-medication use tripled in preschool children ages two to four over a five-year period. These are children in the prime of their mental and physical development, and no studies have been done on the long-term effects of these drugs given to young children.
- The news media is provided with stories designed to create fears about a condition and point out the latest treatment. This leads to: people with normal symptoms taking dangerous drugs, people being tested regularly, and undergoing unnecessary treatments with drugs and invasive surgeries.

People should focus more time and attention on their health as they age or see degeneration starting, rather than settling for a diagnosis and the latest medication. The only winners here are those who profit financially. Even worse, many people passively allow medical intervention for both physical and mental well-being, rather than taking responsibility for their own health and actively participating in it, trusting in the God-given recuperative powers of their body. The result of handing over the responsibility for your health to the medical industrial complex and Big Pharma is that they have become bloated, profitable, and powerful, and people are becoming poorer and sicker.

Not Only Medicine But Also Hospitals Can Be Bad For Your Health

To make things even worse, a stay in the hospital may also contribute to the downward spiral to people's health.

- The most conservative estimate is that between 44,000 and 98,000 Americans die each year from preventable medical care injuries that happen in hospitals. Thus the American hospital is somewhere between the fourth and sixth most common cause of death on the planet. More deaths occur as a result of preventable injuries at hospitals than from the entire AIDS epidemic or from breast cancer each year.

The Healthcare System

- About 40% of a person's total health comes from our behaviors with the three biggest detriments to our health being tobacco, alcohol and other recreational drugs, and obesity. About 30% of our health depends on our genes. About 20% of our health is a result of public health which controls epidemic infectious disease through sanitation and immunization. Only about 10% of our total health comes from the healthcare delivery system, and this year we will spend $6,800 per American on healthcare delivery.

What is our healthcare system trying to accomplish? Is it profit or healthcare? If it is healthcare we would put most of our healthcare money into prevention and primary medical care for everyone. If it is profit, we would minimize prevention and put our efforts into acute care that is needed when prevention is avoided.

The solution is to put the heart back into healthcare. Healthcare should be a shared social benefit for all, and society needs to agree on a basic level of care for everyone. If someone wants to go beyond that and have things that are very expensive or of questionable value, they would need to pay for it. The emphasis should be on preventative care and should offer alternative treatments.

Conclusions

The problem is that healthcare has become a for-profit business with increasing emphasis on ever-increasing profit and thus decreasing emphasis on the ministry of healthcare. The system is corrupt and only a system change will fix the problem.

There are many very good people in healthcare; in fact, I think that healthcare tends to attract those who really want to minister to and serve others for their good. The current situation in healthcare is very frustrating and stressful to most healthcare workers.

Healthcare should be a shared social responsibility, not a profit center. Decisions need to be based on what is needed for all. How can resources be used to treat the many, rather than make the few rich?

The healing professions are one of the highest callings on the planet due to the ministry of one soul to another. That is where true healing occurs. It is a sign of our times that this noble profession is being transformed into an industry for profit. So many people are drawn to the healing professions because they truly want to minister to others, but the current system has become so distorted and corrupted with greed that it is difficult to practice the ministry of healing rather than becoming a part of the medical industrial complex. Love heals, and although there is certainly a place for emergency medicine, antibiotics, and lifesaving surgeries, the current emphasis on fixing emotional problems or conditions that arise from poor nutrition and lack of good health habits with the latest pill is a destructive, non-healing approach.

We live in an era expecting immediate results from our smallest efforts. We are on a road that is leading away from true healing. It is a road that relieves people of their own responsibility for their health through healthy spiritual, mental, emotional, and physical habits. It is a road leading to dependency on corporations that may not have our best interest at heart. It is a road that makes promises that it can't keep and that leads away from the real road to healing that is alignment with divine purpose and brotherly/sisterly love and compassion.

Let's be honest: who makes money if people are healthy? And who makes money when people are sick (or think they are)? Has anyone noticed that we refer to the medical insurance *industry* and the pharmaceutical *industry* rather than the medical insurance *ministry* or pharmaceutical *ministry*? Think about it.[1]

Dr. Marayeh Cunningham is a clinical psychologist and Executive Director of the Soulistic Medical Institute in Tubac, Arizona and Soulistic Hospice in Tubac and Tucson, Arizona.

My Fellow Doctors And Patients The World Over, Mortal Strugglers All, Let Us Unite In The Universal Health-Giver of All—God— For Goodness' Sake

by Landau Lawrence, M.D.

PREFACE: From a doctor's perspective, I heartily thank any patient or their friends and family for trying to make sense about healthcare and money matters which I have struggled professionally for more than thirty years now to better grasp and deal with. I can tell you that I have found that the main trouble we have is that MONEY AND MEDICINE DON'T MIX. They simply can't. So, in that sense alone you are quite right to wish for, and believe in, a world where the money lenders and venders have absolutely no authority whatsoever in health matters.

From a patient's perspective, I can say that the love and care of healing is indeed free, but in order for the gift to translate into its full healing power, it must be qualified through certain attitudes and actions on the part of the afflicted and/or their guardians. There is a price after all: the desire to change, faith, and gratitude. So the solution for the doctors and patients alike, who will ultimately find themselves as one and the same, is to accept God and His healing and then "pay it forward "in the high spirit of, "Freely you have received, freely give!"

My dear friends and fellow occupants and custodians of this Earth, for me there can be no doubt about it: I am a mortal struggler. I've known that I was a struggler in this mortal life for as far back as I can remember. That is to say, I know that I have managed to struggle this whole lifetime over, in good times and in bad, in sickness and in health. And I know that I still do struggle on. And I believe that everyone enshrouded in flesh today is a mortal struggler, to some degree. That means to me that no matter what side of any fence any and all of us may erect, we all share in a common problem, namely mortality.

And we each share a common solution to that common problem. I believe that once more of us realize that all of us are mortal strugglers, sick children so to speak, we can help one another overcome sickness. Impossible? Maybe not! Far away in time and space? Only if we fail to think more clearly and with greater generosity, or fail to unite with one another in higher goals and aspirations. The point I am trying to make is that it is the state of division from each other and from our Unifying Source—God—that sickens and kills us. I believe that *our hour has come* to throw the shackles of disease off humankind and manifest the day when we can actually fulfill the prophecy made by a poet when he said, "Death, be thou not proud!"

Six Decades Of A Split Mind

It took me every bit of six decades on this planet to finally realize that it is the *split mind* that I and all mortal strugglers have developed that keeps that

Unifying Source and Giver of Life from healing any and all of us. The truth is that I have taken sides so much from the very dawn of my consciousness that I've managed in such a blind and broken state to live mostly under the illusion that I and all of my fellows are actually whole beings who somehow wear out over the years for various unknown reasons.

Now, there was a brief period in my life, mostly because of my exposure to my maternal grandmother, that I conceived that there were actually two kinds of people in this world. To me, the vast majority of people on Earth were just like me, strugglers. But there were others like my maternal grandmother whom I thought of as naturals, people, usually much older, who kept the light of goodness on, often just by their presence. At least that was my impression in my first decade of life as a child awakening to the spiritual resources coming especially from within his own extended family. I can't say that I understood much about my so-called "naturals" in those days, but I was grateful for their presence in my life because they made me feel better about myself and all other strugglers.

In my second decade of life, I grew into a patriot becoming proud of what I sensed was a two-hundred-year American heritage of honorable struggling. I found Patrick Henry's Address to the House in 1775 to be a touching and compelling oration for the struggle for freedom over tyranny, but it also introduced a growing concern in my soul that even the best of our world's heroes could themselves be diseased, at least to some extent, by a split mind. For example, Patrick Henry closed his speech with the words, "Give me liberty or give me death," but much of the speech had laced within it the more worrisome message of: "Give me liberty or give YOU death."

The closest American president to becoming a "natural" in my lifetime was John F. Kennedy. I was barely fourteen years old when I watched Kennedy give his Inaugural Address, and my desire to be a world champion soared to new heights when I heard him say: "My fellow citizens of the world: ask not what America will do for you, but what together we can do for the freedom of man." His closing line reached into my deepest desire for godly patriotism. Said he: "With a good conscience our only sure reward, with history the final judge of our deeds, let's go forth to lead the land we love, asking His blessing and His help knowing that here on earth God's work must truly be our own."

Even today, after having fought for, and been mortally wounded, in the pursuit of the kind of citizenship that Kennedy proposed, I am still poised for Kennedy's "my-fellow-citizens-of-the-world" outlook. After all, Kennedy had just identified for all of us, on both sides of any battlefield what our common enemies were: "tyranny, poverty, disease, and war itself." And so to this very day I do remain prepared to rally with the rest of the honest strugglers of the world for actualizing the global yes to his proposal of 1961: "Can we forge against these enemies a grand and global alliance, North and South, East and West, that can assure a more fruitful life for all mankind? Will you join in that historic effort?"

But even in that great speech Kennedy had said something which was worrisome for me. He had said: "For only when our arms are sufficient beyond doubt can we be certain beyond doubt that they will never be used." That didn't ring true at all, and it certainly was out of alignment with Jesus' warning that "Everyone who lives by the sword will die by the sword." For whom, I still wonder, had Kennedy added those words to his speech, for those were words which somehow threatened to undo his entire proposal? Only later did I discover that even Kennedy was held hostage by certain dishonest strugglers, and Kennedy himself ultimately lost his life to the ones who insisted that he carry a sword.

In my third decade of life, I was a soldier and I too carried a sword, meant to defend the good part of Kennedy's proposal, but in fact feeding the common enemies of man, and serving dishonest strugglers like those who had eliminated Kennedy and hidden behind his honor. It wasn't until shortly before I myself was wounded in combat that I realized that I was actually honoring the unhonorable and serving the opponents of our Creator and the Giver of All Life. I actually tried to rectify my errors by going to medical school and learning the healing trade. But my split brain made me and my best intentions vulnerable to the vendors of darkness on this world.

It didn't take me long to discover that the medical associations and pharmaceuticals were all corrupted by the first two letters in sick, S-I, for Self-Interest. In my split-brain blindness, I actually thought I was "doing my part" to fight the organized crime of money-driven medicine until I finally realized that I was no more than an independent criminal myself. What I mean by that is, as a *private practitioner* serving a chosen segment of the population for a certain price, I couldn't see that I was still serving the very disease that dishonest strugglers were using to keep themselves growing in power. Even after I discovered that huge flaw in my thinking, it took me three more decades to turn the misguided train of a split-brain around. Why?

The World Needs More Naturals

I am a mortal struggler whose deep ignorance of my own faults and carelessness has kept me from seeing a window of opportunity in a tunnel of darkness. The world needs more naturals, whom I now think of as the ones who have already found themselves diseased by the Self-Interest Lord and have managed to re-create a new "Age of Innocence." But their re-created Age of Innocence is not the state of naivety; it is a new form of wisdom. It is the global alliance of humility and benevolence, practiced in an atmosphere of the gentle, kind way, void of conceit, rejoicing in hope and patient in tribulation. It is a place where we, the citizens of Earth, conclude that caring for everyone and everything in creation is our calling, and sincerely living that level of caring is our ticket to real, global, universal health.

Once a sufficient number of us are devoted to being completely trustworthy in such a cause of care, then we can find all those others seeking to extend the same quality of care as well, and join forces with them. For earnest, trustworthy care is truly contagious where there is a desire to be a clean servant of others, and being clean of desire and action, it bonds with terrific power to its allies to make new and wonderful alloys of goodness and well-being.

Fellow strugglers of the world, let us dare to care in a completely clean fashion, and let us not allow any of the contaminants of self-interest such as fear, anger, envy, jealousy, suspicion, or intolerance keep us from the bonding health of caring and serving one another. True healing is not about just your health or my health. Neither is it about the absolute avoidance of pain or suffering, since both can be features of growth and repair, and the healthy metamorphosis of cells and tissues into their higher state. Rather, true healing is about the restoration of health and fulfillment for the whole world, and everything and everyone in it.

We do not need all those new and better machines with which to diagnose and treat diseases! We need to let our Creator have His place back in creation and inventions, starting with ourselves, so that all that is and everyone in it can have life and have it more abundantly! We need to come to understand that the kingdom referred to by Jesus is one of purpose in life, artful living, actualized destiny, and all of humanity united in a true brotherhood and sisterhood.

So, instead of putting what can be transient, even perishable, such as physical health, as our highest request of God, let us do what Jesus commanded us to do some two thousand years ago: "Put our minds first on the kingdom of heaven, and all these things are ours without the asking."

Dr. Landau Lawrence is the Medical Director for the Soulistic Medical Institute and Soulistic Hospice.

Hospice—A Winning Situation
by Aládi Goodman, R.N., CHPN

I am a registered nurse and have worked full-time for several years in the field of home hospice care. Hospice care involves caring for terminally-ill individuals, focusing on giving comfort care, which includes relief of pain and other uncomfortable symptoms, as opposed to giving curative care, which involves attempts at curing the patient of a particular illness.

The philosophy behind hospice care is to provide not only for the physical needs of the patient, but also addresses the spiritual, psychosocial, and emotional needs of both the patient and the family/caregiver. Hospice nursing, therefore, is holistic and requires flexibility and the ability to multitask and blend into various roles, as well as being a strong patient advocate and working closely with other members of the Interdisciplinary Team.

Hospice care also places an emphasis on keeping the patient at home with family and friends for as long as possible and has a multidisciplinary team available to meet the needs of the patient and family. This team consists of not only nurses, but physicians, social workers, spiritual-care coordinators/chaplains, certified nursing assistants (CNAs), dieticians, physical/speech/occupational therapists, bereavement counselors, and various volunteer services to name a few. Many hospices also incorporate alternative therapies such as massage, Reiki, acupuncture, music, and pet therapy.

Although I have worked in many different fields of nursing, due to this holistic philosophy and the sense of dignity it brings to patients and their family members, as well as the right to fully participate in their final stage of life, I personally have found home hospice nursing to be the most rewarding so far.

People often ask me how I cope with being around dying people all the time. I share that most often what I experience is very special and uplifting. I also share that I see hospice nursing as being a form of midwifery; however, the transition phase is at the other end of the spectrum of life. I am also personally devoted to a spiritual path and know without a doubt that the person I am caring for is graduating to a higher plane. Sometimes I feel that moving on from this world can actually be a blessing in many ways, especially if the physical body is no longer able to function without pain and suffering, and the person's quality of life is limited. If I am at ease and have complete faith in the dying process and the eternal ascension plan, then this helps the family to be more at peace also.

I have worked within the healthcare system since I was seventeen years old and trained as a nurse in my home country of New Zealand which has socialized medicine. Moving to the U.S. and learning of its healthcare system was a culture shock and challenging in many ways. Having now experienced both forms of healthcare firsthand, I do, without a doubt, think that socialized medicine is a much higher form of healthcare, although it is not perfect.

In New Zealand, I was never concerned about having the finances to meet any of my health needs. I was provided for by the government of my country. I often recall the time when the New Zealand government tried to start billing its citizens to stay in the hospital. The charge was a mere $50 per night, a fraction of what it costs in the USA; however, the people of New Zealand refused to pay, so that went nowhere.

Hospice care in the United States is the closest philosophy I have found yet to incorporating the sense of socialized medicine. If you have a loved one who is dying or has an incurable illness, you can find a hospice that will care for that person, regardless of the patient's ability to pay. Hospice care in the U.S. is usually funded by Medicare, Medicaid, and private insurances; however, there are some individuals who either do not qualify for or cannot afford any of these benefits. I personally have cared for many of these individuals who received the same care as all our patients, regardless of their ability to pay. Is this not how all people should be treated—always, and not only when they are dying?

Various studies show that hospice patients live an average of twenty-nine days longer than similar patients who do not choose hospice care. This can be due to several factors. Firstly, hospice surrounds the patient with compassionate care and support, which is especially important for those without family involvement. For example, those alone in a nursing home—feeling lonely, tired, and hopeless—who suddenly start receiving the loving visits from hospice-care professionals, may find their quality of life enhanced, bringing them hope and renewed energy. Secondly, hospice provides quality and consistent medical care—a hospice nurse can detect medical issues, such as simple infections, that can eventually lead to life-threatening situations, even causing a patient to die prematurely.

Hospice is also an alternative to aggressive treatments such as chemotherapy, radiation, and major surgeries which I have often observed cause further debilitation and decline in a person already compromised from their disease process. Oncologists are trained to treat a cancer aggressively and often will continue to do so right until a person begins to actively die, at which point hospice is called in. I personally have experienced many of these patients dying within the first three days of admission to hospice care and their last round of chemotherapy and/or radiation. Hospice is a gentler alternative approach, treating uncomfortable symptoms only, giving patients the opportunity to live each day out to their fullest potential without any of the side effects that chemotherapy or radiation bring, leaving more energy to devote to their families and the type of interests that enhance their quality of life.

Considering that the most money spent on healthcare is within a person's last year of life, it is a fact that hospice actually is more cost effective. A report out of Duke University (published in *Social Science & Medicine*, 2007) indicated that the use of hospice reduced Medicare costs an average of $2,309 per hospice user in this last year of life. The maximum reduction per hospice user was around $7,000 when the patient had terminal cancer and used hospice for the last 58–103 days of life.

Hospice is definitely a winning situation for all involved. As previously touched upon, I have not experienced this in any other field of nursing I have worked in as of yet, and there have been many. I cannot count the times when I have gone to a person's house to find a very desperate situation of an elderly spouse trying to care for his or her wife or husband alone, not knowing what to do, and being unable to afford a nursing home or private caregivers. I have been able to deliver the good news that help has just arrived, and they need not be alone anymore. I inform them that a licensed nurse can visit them as often as needed, the CNA can take over the bathing of the patient, and we will bring in medical equipment, comfort medications, and supplies, as well as the hospice physician and all those on the Interdisciplinary Team plus more, and they do not personally have to pay a thing. They will even have a nurse available to them on call, 24 hours a day seven days per week.

People just are not used to this type of stress-free, service-oriented treatment from the healthcare system and often will weep tears of joy and relief and treat me as if God just sent in an angel. This is a wonderful experience, but I personally find an aspect of this very sad too. Recently after I had been to a house and experienced this very type of situation, and left after receiving the tears and hugs of relief from an elderly wife who could no longer care for her husband, I went and sat in my car and simply wept.

Why should this kind of help be such a miracle to people, and why shouldn't people expect the very best out of their healthcare system? How can our current healthcare system possibly enhance the healing process? Something is very wrong with this picture, and I look forward to the day when all people, of all races, ages and socioeconomic backgrounds can receive quality healthcare for free, and not just in the last six months of their life—that point when the government and insurance companies have calculated that money will be saved by making such a wonderful service available.

Aládi Goodman is Director of Clinical Services for Soulistic Hospice.

The Gesundheit! Hospital Project
by Patch Adams, M.D.

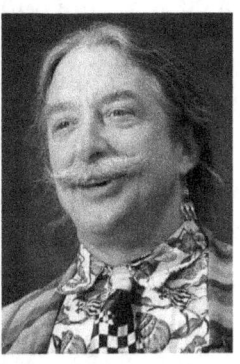

I entered medical school in 1967 to use medicine as a vehicle for social change. I used my free time to study the history of healthcare delivery around the world and to look at contemporary models with the idea of creating a medical model that would address all the problems of the way care is delivered. I didn't intend to create a model that would be the answer to the problems; but to model creative problem solving, and to spark each medical facility to design their own ideal rather than succumb to the garbage of managed care, or a resignation to the impossibility of humanistic care.

Beginning in the climate of the political "war on poverty," I felt confident that a free hospital to serve the poorest state, West Virginia, would find easy funding and that we would be built in four years. I smile writing this as we enter our thirty-third year without having broken ground on the hospital. However, we have asked our architect to go to finished drawings so that we can begin building as soon as we have funding in hand. None of the journey has gone as I imagined and the vision is so much deeper, more comprehensive and far-reaching as a consequence of such deliberate progress.

The original vision had all the principles we have maintained all these years. There would be no charge for the care. Barter was also not an option. In fact, we wanted to eliminate the idea of debt in the medical interaction as a way to begin recreating human community. We didn't want people to think they owed something; we wanted them to think they belonged to something. We could not conceive of a community that did not care for its people. This also meant a refusal to accept third-party reimbursement, both to refuse payment and to sever the stranglehold that insurance companies had on how medicine was practiced. We would have nothing to do with malpractice insurance, which forces fear and mistrust into every medical interaction. We espouse the politics of vulnerability and are clearly aware that we can only offer caring and never promise curing. In such a flagrantly imperfect science, we need the right to make mistakes.

The loudest cry of patients was for compassion and attention, which was a call for time. So initial interviews with patients were three to four hours long, so that we could fall in love with each other. Intimacy was the greatest gift we could give them, especially at a death bed, with intractable pain or chronic, unsolved medical problems. It was natural to insist on a house call to sweeten this intimacy. When I made a house call, I opened every drawer and snooped in every closet. I wanted to know the patients in all of their complexities. An apparent secret in the practice of medicine (so easily erased when business is the context) is how care is bidirectional.

My mother had a below-knee amputation as a result of having diabetes and smoking all of her life. When she was regaining consciousness in Recovery Unit, I smiled at her and said 'Well mum, how does it feel to have one foot in the grave?' She laughed out loud. 'Til the day she died, she told that story to her friends and each time she laughed again.

Patch Adams

This intimacy is as important for the care giver as it is the patient. The bidirectionality of healing is at the core of preventing burnout. The business of medicine has connected the word "care" with the concept "burden," to describe all who need care, who are not wealthy. But we found the unencumbered practice of medicine is an ecstatic experience.

In spending this amount of time with patients, we found that the vast majority of our adult population does not have a day-to-day vitality for life (which we would define as good health). The idea that a person was healthy because of normal lab values and clear x-rays had no relationship to who the person was. Good health was much more deeply related to close friendships, meaningful work, a lived spirituality of any kind, an opportunity for loving service, and an engaging relationship to nature, the arts, wonder, curiosity, passion and hope. All of these are time-consuming, impractical needs. When we don't meet these needs, the business of high-tech medicine diagnoses mental illness and treats with pills.

What the majority need is an engagement with life. This is why we fully integrated medicine with performing arts, arts and crafts, agriculture, nature, education, recreation, and social service, as essential parts of healthcare delivery. We knew that the best medical thing we could do for the patients was to help them have grand friendship skills and find meaning in their lives. This is a major reason that the staff's home was the hospital. We insisted on friendships with our patients (made easy by not charging, and giving them our lives). A patient ideally would bring their whole family while they were healthy, and stay a few days as friends, becoming familiar with the hospital (home, sanctuary), so that just being there was relaxing, even healing.

We wanted patients to bring all their interests and skills to essentially become temporary staff as well as patients during their stay. For example, if a car mechanic came as a patient, we could notify the poor in our greater community who might need their car fixed, and have it happen while the mechanic was getting care. The mechanic may also give classes on basic mechanics. All these features help build community, creating a sense of interdependence. Those receiving care cannot feel indebted because they become both the help and the helped.

To help promote diversity and truly to be full service in our planned facility, we insist on integrating all the healing arts. Allopathic medicine, including surgery, ob/gyn, pediatrics, internal medicine, family practice, and psychiatry, will work hand in hand with complementary medicine, including acupuncture, homeopathy, naturopathy, chiropractic, ayurvedic, anthroposophic, herbal, body work, and faith healing. It will be an exciting opportunity to study how they can all work together under close observation. The entire environment will be an example of preventive medicine exploring how to help a patient and their family grow healthy (or at least healthier!).

From the beginning, social, environmental, and global health were felt to be essential as part of our medicalpractice. There, violence and injustice became medical issues. Unemployment, the discrepancies between rich and poor, poverty, pollution, corrupt governments, and economic systems all become concerns of a medical practice. There was always an invitation and encouragement to become involved in social change, even if the individual did not feel it affected their life. We want to build a fine community of people whose ethic is caring for all. Now, we have added to our vision a school to teach social change with the whole community as its laboratory. Agriculture will not just be about feeding people, but an exploration into sustainable agriculture. We'll use designing the community as an experiment in appropriate technology.

One of the most radical parts of the vision was that we wanted all of the activity to be infused with fun. I wanted to build the first silly hospital in history. Foolishness was embraced, often to extreme, in even the most profound of situations. We had fun deaths and bizarre, outlandish behaviors with the mentally ill. In our normal, serious world with somber medical environments (even though no research supports being serious and thousands of research papers encourage joy and humor as healing), we saw no contradiction in feeling that a hospital could also be an amusement park, even implying it is important for staff and patient.

The ideal staff people we looked for were, by intention, happy, funny, loving, cooperative, and creative. I knew the key to the creation of this beautiful model was in the people deciding and choosing to live there; because it is people that really make a model. Ideas can only be as real as the people living them. Politically, our most potent wedge for change would be living happily together, in constant, joyful service, fully expressing our creative selves at extremely low salaries. The point was not to try to teach a staff this, but to find people for whom this was their way of life.

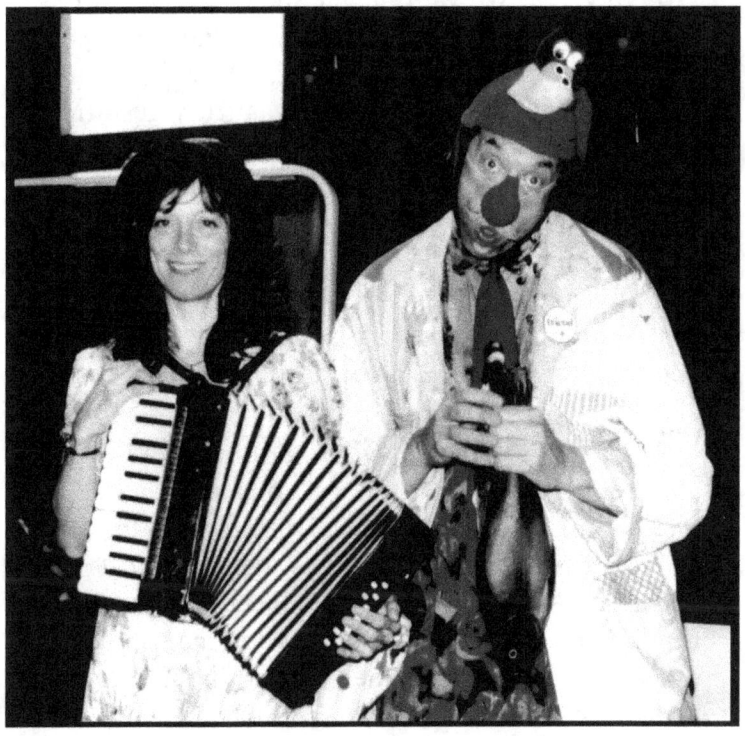

Patch Adams and Susan Parenti in Cuba
source: http://patchadams.org

In our first twelve years (1971–1983) we did all this as a pilot project. Twenty adults and our children moved into a large, six-bedroom house and called ourselves a hospital. We were open twenty-four hours a day, seven days a week, for all manner of medical problems from birth to death. Three of the adults were physicians. We saw 500–1000 people each month, with five to fifty overnight guests a night; totaling 15,000 people over those twelve years. We were never sued. At least three thousand of the patients had mental illness, and we did not give psychiatric medicines. We referred out what we could not handle. It was truly ecstatic, fascinating, and stimulating. No one gave us a donation and we were 0:1400 for foundation grants, so our staff had to work part-time jobs to pay to practice medicine. After nine years of nobody leaving, most staff said they felt we would never be funded and wanted to stop. It was the saddest moment for me, for I loved all of them and knew that I had to persevere.

I tried to recreate the work for three more years and realized that in order to continue, I need a facility to support this model of care. Now the job was to raise the funds to build it. It appeared that our ideas were too radical to get conventional funding, and so I realized that we had to go to the people of the world to get the needed funds. The model for that in modern society is through publicity and fame. So I broke a basic tenet of our philosophy, no publicity, and became public. For the last twenty years we have climbed that fame and fortune ladder in hopes that we would attract funds to build our ideal rather than compromise the vision. This went to monstrous extremes in 1998 when a feature film, Patch Adams, was released with Robin Williams playing me.

These efforts have brought us a 317-acre farm in Pocahontas County, West Virginia. The land has three waterfalls, with caves behind one. We built a four-acre pond, there is a mountain of hardwood trees and twenty-eight acres of rich bottom land that has had no chemicals on it for twenty-two years. We have built two beautiful buildings in anticipation of someday building the hospital. Two years ago, with a little sadness that the hospital was still not built, and a hunger to begin seeing patients again, I agreed to consider reopening with a first phase that would include an outpatient clinic and a school for social change, with residence facilities for the staff. We have asked our architect of twenty-one years to give us finished drawings for it. We owe no money and have a good start for Phase 1.

I could feel frustrated, even sad, that the hospital is still unbuilt. However, in the long run it may prove to have been a very positive time line. After thirty-three years, we have built a much larger, more diverse, more intelligent, more globally influential model than we ever dreamed of in those first twelve incubating years. Our global impact has affected far more patients' lives and inspired more social change than if we had gotten our funding early on. My failure at fundraising has forced me and our evolutionary staff and friends to expand in every direction and meet a quality and quantity of people that make our greater team of friends and contacts number in the thousands in almost every area of endeavor, especially healing, the arts, and social change. Gesundheit! has indeed become a global mover and shaker active in forty or more countries, expanding beautifully all the time.

When we build the model with people serving it, full and part time, its example will be breathtaking with a process already in place to have an important impact because a variation of that is happening already. The patients of our first twelve years were individuals and families looking closely at their organ systems. The patients of our last twenty years have been communities and societies looking at their organ systems: environmental, social, political, economic. All of these "patients" will dance through the hospital when it is built. I have had to earn the funds to support these last twenty years' activities, with every month being a creative journey of survival.

Since the film's release, we're not on such a survival edge, but we have still not raised funds for major construction. The beauty of the journey makes patience easy, especially since every day is wildly exciting and globally influential, regardless of the building progress. This is not to say that the building of the hospital is any less important. On the contrary: it is more important than ever since it has remained, these thirty-one years, the only model in the U.S. (and one of few in the world) to comprehensively address healthcare delivery problems. Our example of joyful persistence alone is an important, inspiring model for the changes needed in the world.

We stopped seeing patients in 1983 to devote ourselves to fundraising full time for the hospital, by expanding out into the world. I began lecturing and performing on a wide variety of subjects (fifty lectures, shows and workshops) with every imaginable kind of audience and with as many as eleven lectures in a day. All levels of education from elementary schools to medical schools (most of the ones in the United States and in thirty to forty countries), churches, community centers, conferences, and corporations. For most of the time it was for 150–200 days a year and 300 days a year since the film, always all over the world. A constant flow of publicity and my two books translated into ten languages and the film have made our project part of the medical dialogue all over the world when referring to humanized health care.

During these twenty years our clown healing work has expanded all over the world, so that clowns are now a regular part of hospitals on every continent, and this is expanding as people hear the message that it is really about spreading joy in every public space as gestures toward peace, justice, and care. I started taking clowns to prisons, foreign countries, even to refugee camps, and war zones. For eighteen years I've taken thirty clowns from all over the world to Russia for two weeks of clowning in hospitals, orphanages, prisons, and nursing homes, as well as airports, subways, streets, and hotels.

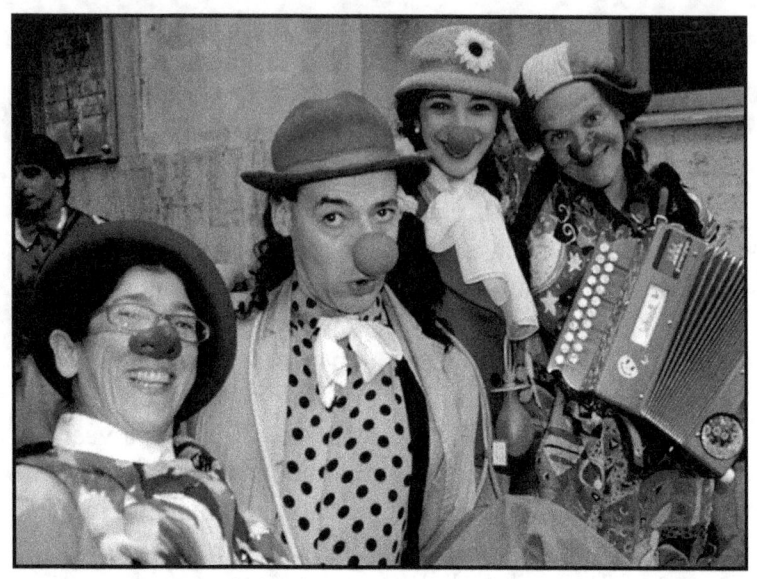

Gesundheit! clowns in Argentina

source: http://patchadams.org

Ten years ago this led to our getting involved in the care of orphans in Russia in work that is now recognized all over. We have taken clowns into the war in Bosnia, the Kosovo refugee camps in Macedonia, the Rumanian AIDS orphanages, African refugee camps, Cuba, China, El Salvador, Korea, and Haiti. As I write this, we took twenty-two clowns from all six continents and ten tons of aid for three and a half weeks into the war in Afghanistan. Because this work has connected us with many aid and relief organizations (like Airline Ambassadors), it is now easy to organize huge quantities of people and aid quickly and effectively.

These experiences have also gotten us involved in the global conversations on conflict resolution.

All of our gestures of love and fun have been a magnet for beautiful people who want to devote their lives to loving service. Every year thousands of doctors and nurses tell me they would be willing to live and work full time 40 to 60 hour weeks in our hospital for $3,000/year. Many more want to come part time. Students of medicine from all over the world constantly entreat us to let them come study what we are doing. This may be the most important reason to get the hospital built.

Nine years ago a special group of old and new friends began to come together in a real group commitment toward the dream; our second major staff change. No longer did I have to carry the vision alone because the individuals of this group—though quite diverse in thought and personality—each felt they found a place and readiness in themselves to want to be and work for the now-collective vision. For any project created by one person this is a grand step so that the vision can continue if something happens to the visionary. Another important bonus is that each of them brings their special interests and talents to the project to vastly broaden how the multiple tasks I used to do now get done, and each adds their blessed creativity again enhancing every part of the vision. What it feels like to me is that now everything is in place to make the hospital a reality.

We plan to build a forty-bed rural community hospital. There will be sixty beds for staff and beds for their families in a creative, comfortable communal hospital. There will also be forty beds for guests who would be healing arts students on electives, ophthalmology teams every three months, plumbers, string quartets, and anyone wanting a service-oriented vacation. There will be 30,000 square feet devoted to the arts in a fully arts-centered hospital. There will be a school for social change and in-depth agricultural programs. It will be funny looking, full of surprises and magic. We'll be exploring how far below the national average our effective operating budget can run. I believe we'll be shockingly inexpensive. Our ideal is that an endowment would cover the annual costs and realize without this we'll find creative ways to pay for its operation.

There will be a forty-acre village to house our children's school (also for sick children and children of sick parents) and other important community experiments, like how to integrate all ages in a fun, healthy way. Staff persons who've served for four years and want a little distance from the intensity of the hospital can create their fantasy living space in our village.

I want to tell all readers that the journey has been heavenly all along the way. Simply being in an idealist quest is its own reward. I've never felt I've sacrificed anything or thought it was a hard journey. Hard would have been having to work in corporate medicine and lie to patients and myself every day. My concern for humanity's future drives me to want to put whatever efforts I can to changing everything that hurts people and nature. The Gesundheit! Institute is that for me, and so many others.

Patch's Prescription:
10 Everyday Actions to Help Heal Society

1. Pick up all the trash in an area in your hometown; be its guardian. Tell others about it.
2. Be friendly to every one at all times; experiment outrageously.
3. Offer a shoulder or foot rub in any environment.
4. Always speak up for justice, no matter how much it costs.
5. Go once a week on a "house call" to a nursing home to cheer people up as a friend.
6. Turn off your TV and become interesting. Perform yourself.
7. Consider being silly in public. Sing out loud. Wear funny stuff.
8. Find ways to need a whole lot less money; share beyond belief.
9. Have potlucks frequently, with neighbors, co-workers, strangers. Work toward living in extended families.
10. Take your vacations in your own hometown and spend the money working on projects there that help build community.

source: http://patchadams.org

Attention movie stars, sports stars, rock stars, surgeon stars (including other doctors who have tons of money in the bank and wish you were doing what Patch is doing but are not brave enough to do it, because of course you don't want to "damage" your reputation), and all millionaires and billionaires:

Please help Patch build his hospital by giving generously of your excess finances to this most valuable and much-needed cause.

— Gabriel of Urantia

For more information:
http://patchadams.org

Patch Adams does not use email, but he personally answers all regular mail sent to:
Gesundheit Institute
P.O. Box 307
Urbana, IL 61803 USA
Fax: (208) 323-0848

Make Donation Checks Payable to:
Gesundheit! Institute
P.O. Box 50104
Arlington, VA 22205 USA

Gesundheit is a 501(c)(3) tax-exempt organization.

Fundraising contacts only,
call: (217) 278-3933 ext. 12, or
email: giving@patchadams.org

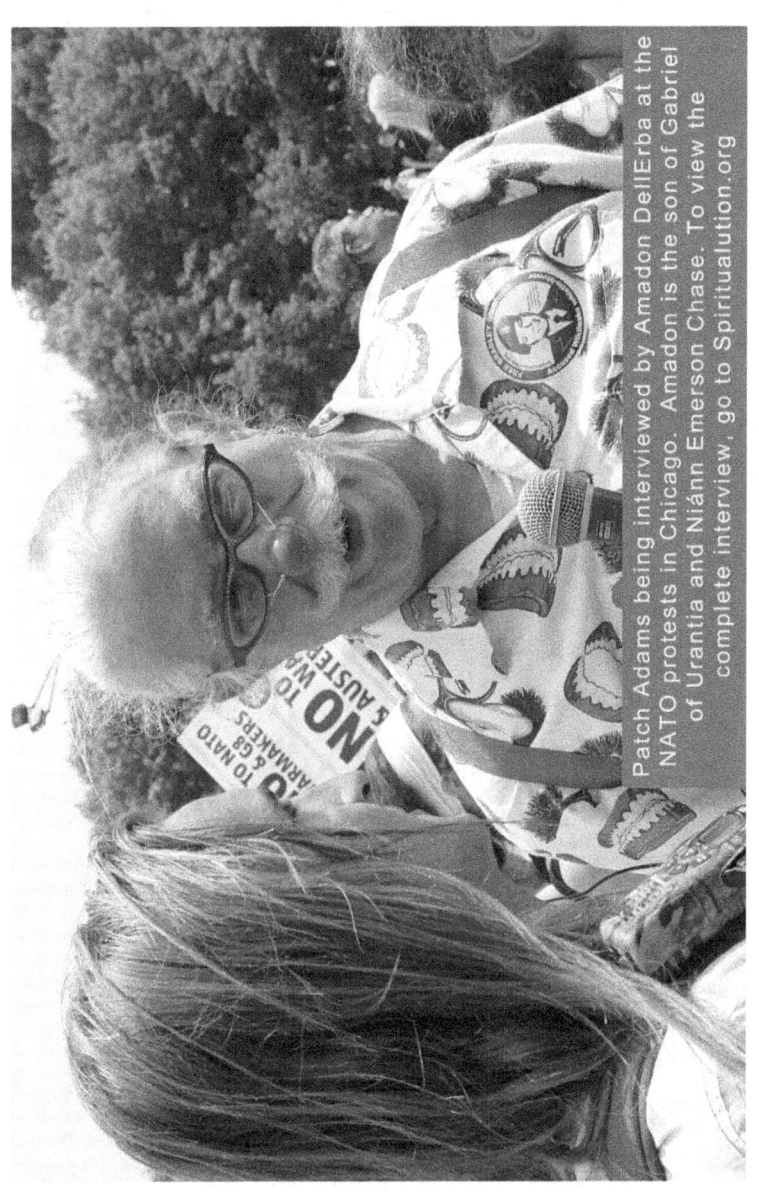

Patch Adams being interviewed by Amadon DellErba at the NATO protests in Chicago. Amadon is the son of Gabriel of Urantia and Niánn Emerson Chase. To view the complete interview, go to Spiritualution.org

Pills

by Minister LaTaYea Calviero

We live
in a society
that has a pill for everything.

In fact,
as of late,
the commercials on TV
seem to be
creating
new diseases,
just so you can buy the pill
that promises
the cure.

Sadly,
our last few
generations
have been trained
since childhood
to reach
for the medicine cabinet
at the first signs
of discomfort.

We've become
dependent
on drugs
—synthetic compounds—
to seemingly
fix biological, physiological,
and psychological things.

Then,
if
the over-the-counter
stuff
doesn't do the trick
quick
enough,
well a pricey visit
to see the doctor
and some
even pricier
prescriptions
will surely fix everything
they claim.

By the time
you ingest
enough pills,
there's NO chance
you'll really get to see

or experience
the symptoms
(albeit with some discomfort)
that may be
a cry for help
from the body
at a much deeper level.

We've been trained
to stop pain
at all costs,
even if the pain
had a message for us,
something to teach us,
to compel us to look further
and find the real solutions
to some of our problems—
and not just the physical problems
of life.

To worsen matters,
the powers that be
have stripped the nutrition
out of our foods and
the earth and her soils,
and then
these same evil souls
have the audacity

to sell us back
the very nutrients
they took away
in the guise of
supplements and vitamins.

Ahhh, more pills.

What ever happened
to eating right?
What ever happened
to good nutrition,
from fresh foods?
And sunshine
and friendship
and solid families?

And what ever happened
to the power of prayer
and rest,
and faith,
and trust,
and nature,
and patience,
and peace?
You know, that peace that passes all
understanding?

I can understand,
in my own struggles
at times,
the desire
that wells up
so strongly
for an "instant fix"—
something to stop
the pain or discomfort
(physical or emotional)
right away
because it seems
like I just
can't take
another second of it all.

But as a dear friend
recently
said to me,
"Peace doesn't come in a pill."

And ya know,
neither does
faith,
or trust,
or maturity,
or love
or true healing
of any kind.

Some things you have to work at,
the old-fashioned way:
one day at a time,
in the company of others,
and with the hand of God.

Of course,
probably any day now
the pharmaceutical industry
will market
a new "Peace Pill".

I can just see the advertising everywhere:
The new F.D.A.-approved
"Instant Nirvana Pill—
Take two
and you won't need
to call us in the morning!"

I say,
"Take 5
(5 minutes that is),
and go talk to God."

I think His idea of Nirvana
is a little different.
And
I'm sure
it doesn't come in a pill.

Soulistic Medical Institute — A Nonprofit Organization

by Marayeh Cunningham, Ph.D., Clinical Psychologist

In order for the body to truly heal, the soul must heal. At the Soulistic Medical Institute we understand the key role each patient plays in his or her own healing process and the importance of a wholehearted desire to heal holistically, or rather soulistically. We endeavor to foster true health, not just absence of disease. We work with individuals of all ages and in all stages of disease and healing.

With this philosophy in mind, the members of the healing team at the Soulistic Medical Institute are trained to discern the root cause of illness-whether physical, emotional, or spiritual. We work as a team of professionals, for we understand the interdependence of the various body systems and the related interdependent treatment methods that may be needed. Soulistic Medicine addresses the person and the person's environment as a whole.

The Soulistic Medical Institute is located in Tubac, Arizona. We offer integrative medical services and are expanding our services to include hospice and palliative care. Much of our healing work is done in people's homes, and we believe in treating the whole family when the whole family is affected.

The healing team consists of a physician, clinical psychologist, registered nurses, and massage therapists—all licensed in the state of Arizona—as well as Reiki practitioners. Other spiritual ministers also comprise the healing team. Morontia (soul) Counseling is also available. All of us who are staff members of the Soulistic Medical Institute feel called by God to serve our brothers and sisters. We do not receive financial compensation for our services; we serve out of love and calling. We endeavor to serve all people of all economic levels who have a sincere desire to actively participate in their own healing process. A sliding-scale fee is available to better serve people of various economic levels, and no one is refused service because of an inability to pay.

At the Soulistic Medical Institute a healing plan is designed for each unique soul and implemented with that individual in order to meet his or her needs. This may include Morontia Counseling (a form of psychospiritual counseling), conventional and alternative medicine, and other complementary modalities. When appropriate, spiritual counseling with Gabriel of Urantia, founder of the Soulistic Medical Institute, is available. Additionally, the incorporation of herbal and nutritional advice, and/ or massage and exercise planning may be recommended elements of an individual's healing program. Although most of these services are provided on an out-patient basis, residency programs are also available for more intensive healing purposes.

Healing Versus Curing

Most doctors are in the business of curing, not healing, and they do not deal with the thought processes of the person. Although we at the Soulistic Medical Institute provide curative care for acute and chronic illness with an integrative medical approach, we also work toward true and lasting healing. Physicians attempt to cure; true ministers attempt to bring about healing. Curing has to do with physical symptoms. Healing has to do with psychospiritual growth. Curing deals with the temporary, whereas healing deals with the permanent, the eternal value of the personality and the soul. Healing has to do with a shift in the mind, in the thought processes of the individual. At the Soulistic Medical Institute we practice both curing and healing.

The Healing Process

Health has to do with our relationship with God and our relationships with others and it is within this realm that healing occurs. The power of love to heal is unimaginable. In order for true healing to take place changes in thought patterns, emotional balancing, and physical cleansing must occur so that the mind, emotions, and body can function properly. This involves developing the necessary discipline to change one's thought, emotional, and physical habits in order to be in the will of God.

The first step in the healing process at the Soulistic Medical Institute is to assess the initial changes that need to be made, including identifying the primary soul problems, incorrect thought patterns, emotional imbalances, Father/Mother/Son circuit imbalances, and physical imbalances. A plan is then formulated to correct these problems. This healing plan often includes counseling as the central ingredient, as all change begins in the mind. Due to the extent of misalignment with divine pattern that all inhabitants of this world have experienced, additional services are required to cleanse and nourish the body to begin the process of physical repair necessary. Such complementary services as nutritional and exercise counseling, homeopathic remedies, massage, Reiki, and traditional medicine may be employed to help the body return to its optimal state of health. If such long term misalignment had not occurred, counseling alone would be sufficient to reestablish health. The goal of counseling and work in this area is not just to eliminate disease and symptoms, but to enjoy perfect health and maintain body and soul in the way God intended.

Our healing process is really our ascension process, and each person's process is unique. Recent research is showing that epigenetics are very powerful—meaning our thoughts, attitudes and motivations can actually turn certain genes on and off. In other words, our health is not only dependent on our genetics but also on our thoughts that determine which of our inherited genes will be activated. Thus, thoughts may determine health even more than genetics.

True healing happens on three levels—spiritual, mindal, and physical. Some physical illnesses do have primarily physical causes. However, for many chronic illnesses if just the physical is treated without dealing with the root cause, which is often a soul issue, then the physical may not be healed or another physical problem may occur in another system of the body.

Healing comes from increased consciousness. Morontia Counseling focused on spiritual progress, fulfillment of destiny purpose, and personality actualization results in true healing. Change, whether it be physical, mental, spiritual, emotional, or social, is difficult, and a person will not change unless they are motivated and hungry for change.

Fulfilling our destiny purpose is essential to healing, for no true healing can take place outside of destiny purpose actualization. Healing has to do with meeting one's destiny. We each have a God-given destiny that we are on this planet to fulfill, and healing has to do with the process of coming into alignment with God's blueprint for our life.

Some souls on the planet have had past lives, and for these souls, past life experiences can have an influence on present day reality. The cosmic genetics a person carries is another factor that needs to be taken into consideration in the healing process. People who are interested in exploring the underlying psychospiritual patterns that may be involved in their physical problems may be interested in seeking the healing ministries of the Soulistic Medical Institute.

Soulistic Medical Institute's Core Healing Team

Minister Landau P. Lawrence, M.D. is a general practitioner with more than thirty years experience who specializes in Soulistic Medicine. He delivers traditional western medical care with compassion and spiritual insight. He makes house calls and treats each patient as a unique individual, taking the time necessary to understand and treat the whole person. In addition to the honor and privilege of serving each soul, he feels being a patient's physician carries many responsibilities and that most important of all is the power of caring for and communicating with each and every soul as though God Himself were personally present in the healing effort. Dr. Lawrence believes that this, along with the dedication to be responsible before God moment-to-moment in every decision and exchange, is what a physician should strive for.

Minister Aládi Goodman, RN, CMSRN, CHPN was born and raised in Christchurch, New Zealand and received her diploma as a comprehensive registered nurse in 1993. Her nursing experience includes psychiatric, post-partum, geriatric, rehabilitation, orthopedic, home health, and hospice care. She completed her medical-surgical certification and is also a certified hospice and palliative care nurse. Aládi is sensitive to both patients and family members and has dedicated her life to serving humanity through ministering to the physical and spiritual needs of others.

Minister Beyana Grace, RN graduated with a BSRN from Arizona State University, Tempe in 1980. She has worked in women's health and geriatrics and has done graduate studies in Somatic Psychology/Dance Movement Therapy at Naropa University, Boulder, Colorado. Beyana is a true caregiver in the deepest sense of the word, bringing warmth and God's love to all whose life she touches.

I, **Minister Marayeh Cunningham, Ph.D.**, the author of this article, have been licensed as a psychologist since 1971 and have worked with a wide variety of people in a variety of life circumstances. For more than twenty years my practice has focused on the soul/mind/body connection and fostering spiritual growth. I approach each individual as a unique ascending son or daughter of God and seek to be a vessel through which God can work to bring peace, hope, and comfort to those who need it most.

I am deeply indebted to Gabriel of Urantia and Niánn Emerson Chase for training me as a Morontia Counselor. I have been privileged to study and practice as a student under them for almost twenty-five years, and I recognize and honor them both for their relationship with God which has allowed Continuing Fifth Epochal Revelation to be brought to the planet.

Morontia Counseling

One of the most successful forms of healing is Morontia Counseling, which involves counseling and rehabilitating the soul. The soul may have negative patterns developed in this life or possibly astral patterns which have been displayed over many lifetimes. Since we are what we think, an individual must begin to purify his or her mind circuitry by overcoming negative thought patterns and non-virtuous behavior. Many diseases in the body have root causes in the emotional and astral bodies where a series of negative thought patterns have disrupted the body's systems over a period of time and caused disease. When emotions are imbalanced they can also disrupt relationships and cause actual physical pain to the body.

Morontia Counseling is a form of psychospiritual counseling—an ascension science process involving the relationship between mind and spirit—based on concepts in *The URANTIA Book* (Fifth Epochal Revelation) and *The Cosmic Family* volumes (Continuing Fifth Epochal Revelation). It is a spiritual teaching and counseling process that fosters spiritual growth and healing. Thus true healing of the whole person encompasses many essential elements involving the active participation of the person who needs the healing.

This involves analyzing yourself for harmful mindal and behavioral patterns, admitting and correcting them, and cooperating with the living spiritual forces available to you to accelerate your healing process. All true healing involves the active participation of the patient. Modern healing practices have tended to reduce the effort of the patient, resulting in dependence on the doctor rather than patients taking responsibility for their own healing in partnership with healing professionals.

Hospice

The last phase of life offers some of the greatest opportunities for growth and healing as we let go of the ego trips of this world and embrace larger values and prepare for our birth from this life into the next.

As a baby grows from a single cell into an infant in just nine months, the end of life can provide such a period of rapid spiritual growth and true healing. Mortals are eternal souls, and our healing does not end with our death but continues on the next plane of existence where we take up where we left off.

We embrace the privilege to be a part of this process with humility and deep respect for the individuals and families who allow us to assist and share in this sacred passage of life when a person prepares to graduate from this planet. The Soulistic Medical Institute opened the Soulistic Hospice in the Summer of 2008 and serves all of Santa Cruz County and Southern Pima County from Nogales to Tucson and is located in Tucson and Tubac, Arizona (in an area known for centuries as the "Palm of God's Hand.")

Contact Us

If this approach to healing resonates with you, and you feel you or someone you love would benefit from this approach you can contact the Soulistic Medical Institute at (520) 398-3970 to find out more about our services, or visit us at 26 Tubac Road Suite B, Tubac, Arizona. If you are a healing practitioner who resonates with our philosophy please contact us for more information and explore the possibility of joining our healing team as a member of our staff.

soulisticmedicalinstitute.org
(520) 398-3970

Book Review

*by Minister Lah-May Bremer,
Hospice I.T. Administrator*

Teachings On Healing, From A Spiritual Perspective
by Gabriel of Urantia and Niánn Emerson Chase

In their book, *Teachings On Healing, From A Spiritual Perspective*, Gabriel of Urantia and Niánn Emerson Chase bring new perspectives to the concept of healing. While many see healing as the body being cured of its infirmities, Gabriel of Urantia and Niánn Emerson Chase expand true healing to include mindal and spiritual healing.

In their teachings, the authors address issues that many medical doctors either choose to overlook or lack the experience to deal with. Since they began their work together in 1988—establishing an intentional spiritual community based on Divine Administration—they have, in their teachings and publications, taught that human health and happiness can be affected by soul issues such as self-pity, pride, and anger. The remedies they offer are not necessarily quick fixes, but require the patient to look at and work on their own patterns—patterns that can not only manifest into illness and disease, but also prevent an individual from growing emotionally and spiritually, limiting what they can contribute to their fellow brothers and sisters.

Sharing personal stories, Gabriel of Urantia and Niánn Emerson Chase help the reader understand more deeply the human condition and the uniqueness of each individual's healing process.

There is a science behind healing, and while the patient (and we are all patients on this planet) may not necessarily comprehend all that is involved, one concept that can be understood as being concomitant with healing is that of ascension. As the individual endeavors to make those changes in consciousness, in thought patterns, and truly tunes in to the leadings of the living spiritual forces as to what he or she should do, ascension happens and true healing can follow. As Gabriel of Urantia states, "You cannot continue to be healed of your various maladies unless you continually ascend."

In *Teachings On Healing, From A Spiritual Perspective*, Gabriel of Urantia and Niánn Emerson Chase provide a clearer perspective on what it takes to heal for all types of souls—older starseed souls and younger souls alike. Taken to heart, the teachings in this book will serve as an impetus for introspection and self-evaluation—necessary components to begin the true healing process.

For more information or to purchase please visit:
globalchangetools.org

NOTES

The Sharp End of the Needle

[1] *The American Heritage® Dictionary of the English Language, Third Edition* copyright © 1992 by Houghton Mifflin Company. Electronic version licensed from InfoSoft International, Inc.

Appeal for More Organ Transplant Research and Artificial Organ Transplants

[1] Wikipedia

Eco-Systems, Social-Systems, and Person-Systems

[1] See Paper 2, Section 7, Paragraph 4 and Paper 100, Section 3, Paragraph 7 of *The URANTIA Book*.

[2] Ibid., Paper 76, Section 3, Paragraph 6.

[3] Ibid., Paper 98, Section 2, Paragraph 3.

[4] Ibid., Paper 48, Section 4, Paragraph 6.

[5] Ibid., Paper 160, Section 4, Paragraph 1.

[6] Ibid., Paper 194, Section 3, Paragraph 7.

The Medical Industrial Complex

[1] AMA seeks cure for merger fever. (2007, December 10). *American Medical News*, p. 1.

Angrisano, C., Farrell, D., Kocher, B., Laboissiere, M., & Parker, S. (2007, January). *Accounting for the Cost of Health Care in the United States*. McKinsey & Company.

Ault, A. (2007, December). Merck Offers $4.85 Billion Payout; FDA Reform Underway. *Family Practice News*, p. 6.

Berry, Emily. (2007, December 10). California fines plan for failing to reveal policy cancellation incentive. *American Medical News*, pp. 19–20.

Berry, Emily. (2008, February 18). United Health faces stiff fines in California. *American Medical News*, pp. 30–31.

Bloom, Mark. (2008, February 11). House Committee Cites Emails Suggesting Drug Makers Hid ENHANCE Results. *MedPage Today*. Retrieved February 12, 2008, from http://medpagetoday.com/ProductAlert/Prescriptions/dh/8321.

Borger, J. (2001, February 13). Drug Industry Stalks the U.S. Corridors of Power. *The Guardian*.

Donohue, A. & Gordon, G. (2000, September 29). Congressional Conflicts of Interest. McClatchy Newspapers.

Facts and Stats about the State of American Health Care. (2007, October 21). *The Sedona Observer*. Retrieved February 2, 2008, from http://sedonaobserver.com/HealthFacts.htm

Fee Schedule Survey. (2004-2007). *Physicians Practice*, p. 22.

Financial Barriers. Healthcare: Facing Barriers. The University of Utah. Retrieved February 8, 2008, from http://kued.org/productions/healthcare/barriers/financial.php.

Health Care Costs: A Primer. (2007, August). The Henry J. Kaiser Family Foundation.

Institutional Conflicts-of-Interest Policies Lacking in Many Medical Schools. (2008, February 12). *MedPage Today*. Retrieved February 13, 2008, from http://medpagetoday.com/PublicHealthPolicy/HealthPolicy/dh/8335.

Interview: Brent James, Vice President for Medical Research Intermountain Healthcare. Healthcare: Facing Barriers. The University of Utah. Retrieved February 2, 2008, from http://kued.org/productions/healthcare/interviews/brentJames.php.

Kuehn, B. (2008, January 9/16). FDA's Science Infrastructure Failing. *JAMA*, Vol. 299, No. 2, pp.157–158.

Lloyd-Jones, D., & Greenland, P. (2008, February 27). Critical Lessons from the ENHANCE Trial. *JAMA*, Vol. 200, No. 8, pp. 953–955.

Lurie, P. (2007, November 5). Presentation before the Institute of Medicine Committee on Conflict of Interest in Medical Research, Education, and Practice. HRG Publication #1830. Retrieved January 12, 2008 fromhttp:// citizen.org/publications.

Matthews, Renee. (2008, January 1). Policy & Practice. *Family Practice News*, p. 45.

Neale, T. (2008, January 10). U.S. Health Care Spending Accelerates Slightly. *MedPage Today*. Retrieved January 1, 2008, from http://medpagetoday.com/PublicHealth-Policy/MedicaidMedicare/dh/7923

Peck, P. (2008, April 15). Rofecoxib (Vioxx) Studies on Mortality were Controlled by Drug Company. *MedPage Today*. Retrieved April 16, 2008 from http://medpagetoday.com/Rheumatology/Arthritis/tb/9128.

Phend, C. (2008, January 16). Efficacy Overstated for Antidepressants. *MedPage Today*. Retrieved January 1, 2008, from http://medpagetoday.com/Hematology-Oncology/ClinicalTrials/dh/7977.

Preventing Medication Errors: Quality Chasm Series. (2006, July 20). Institute of Medicine report.

Relman, A. (2007, December 12). Medical Professionalism in a Commercialized Health Care Market. *JAMA*, Vol. 298, No. 22, pp. 2668–2670.

Smith, M. (2008, February 18). FDA Missed Heparin Plant Inspection in China. *MedPage Today*. Retrieved February 19, 2008, from http://medpagetoday.com/ProductAlert/Prescriptions/dh/8402.

Smith, M. (2008, January 31). Iatrogenic Events, Both Benign and Severe, Frequent in Neonatal Unit. *MedPage Today*. Retrieved February 1, 2008, from http://medpagetoday.com/Pediatrics/GeneralPediatrics/dh/8185.

The Future of Drug Safety: Promoting and Protecting the Health of the Public. (2006, September 22). Institute of Medicine report.

The Medicated Child: Interview: Merrill Goozner. (2007, August 18). FRONTLINE Related Pages, from http://pbs.org/wgbh/pages/frontline/medicatedchild/interviews/goozner.html

The Tightening Grip of Big Pharmaceutical Companies. (2001, April 4). *The Lancet*, 357:9263.

About the Author . . .
Gabriel of Urantia

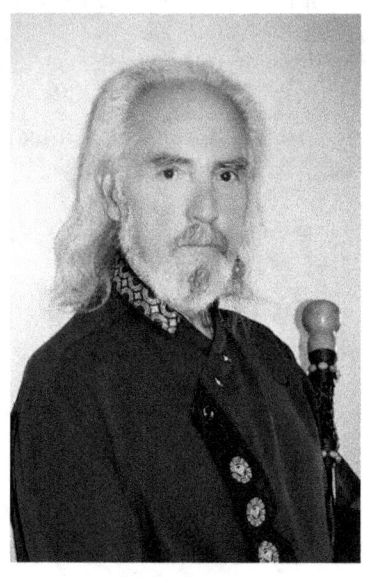

Gabriel of Urantia was born in Pittsburgh, Pennsylvania, where he studied theology at Duquesne University and became one of the first students involved in the charismatic renewal of the Catholic Church, exploring priesthood in Benedictine and Franciscan monasteries in three states. He has worked as an ordained minister and counselor at various spiritual communities across the United States, including the Nicky Cruz/Teen Challenge organization and Youth with a Mission in Hollywood, California.

On the campus of the University of Arizona, he founded a student spiritual organization and became a volunteer chaplain of the Pima County Sheriff's

Department in southern Arizona. For eleven years he worked with the homeless and destitute in his early life, providing shelter and counseling at a halfway house he established on 4th Avenue in Tucson, Arizona, as part of his nonprofit Son Light Ministries. He has been in rehabilitation for 35 years and also started the Personality Integration Rehabilitation Program, now based in Tumacácori, Arizona.

He has explored the writings of all major religions, denominations, and metaphysical sects, progressing on to *The URANTIA Book*.

In 1989 Gabriel of Urantia and Niánn Emerson Chase co-founded Global Community Communications Alliance and Avalon Organic Gardens & EcoVillage, presently based in southern Arizona, in Tubac/Tumacácori. Gabriel and Niánn also co-founded the Soulistic Medical Institute, located in Tubac, Arizona and Soulistic Hospice, located in Tubac and Tucson, Arizona.

Gabriel is a published author (see back of this book), an environmental and social activist, and a spiritual teacher and leader.

Gabriel of Urantia is also an accomplished songwriter/singer/performer. In 1985 he recorded a 33 RPM vinyl vocal spiritual commercial album, *Unicorn Love*, and later introduced another unique style of music, CosmoPop®, to the world, now performing concerts nationwide. You can find his music at globalchangemusic.org

Gabriel of Urantia lives with his present wife, TiyiEndea, and his family of four children at Global Community Communications Alliance at Avalon Organic Gardens & EcoVillage.

Gabriel of Urantia's
SERVICE MINISTRY EXPERIENCE

Duquesne University
Pittsburgh, Pennsylvania

- One of the first students at Duquesne University to be involved in the Charismatic Catholic Renewal, which led to an acquaintance with Maria Von Trapp and daughters (of *The Sound of Music* fame). Agatha Von Trapp became a personal spiritual mentor. A framed letter from her hangs in my office and states:

    > *'Wait on the Lord' is my advice to you and let Jesus handle all your affairs. They could be in no better hands. Wishing you all the blessings of the Lord's resurrection.*
    >
    > **— Agatha Von Trapp**

- Attended Notre Dame University for seminar and convention with 3,000 charismatic priests and 30,000 laymen from all over the world
- Ordained for the first time with United Brethren Evangelical, under Rev. Carlton Pearce
- Attended Catholic charismatic meetings
- Led Bible studies for all denominations within charismatic renewal, student of Rev. Russell Bix
- Wrote articles for a Catholic charismatic magazine, *The Body Builder*

Katherine Kuhlman Ministries
Pittsburgh, Pennsylvania

- Bible student
- Received additional instruction from my personal spiritual advisor, Katherine Kuhlman
- Received certificate of completion for Voice of Prophecy Home Bible Study Course

Hebrew Christian Center (Messianic Jewish Ministry) Pittsburgh, Pennsylvania

- Bible student
- Received additional biblical instruction in Old and New Testaments from my Israeli personal spiritual advisor, Ruth Harris

Holy Trinity Benedictine Monastery
St. Davids, Arizona

- Attended as a brother initiate, under Abbot Father Lewis

Pecos New Mexico Benedictine Monastery
Pecos, New Mexico

- Attended for a several-week study on becoming a spiritual advisor, under Abbot David Garretts
- Studied Jungian psychology and dream analysis

Franciscan Third Order Community
Montrose, Colorado

- Attended Franciscan Third Order Community and first learned of sustainable building and dome construction

Nicky Cruz Organization (Halfway Houses)
Huntington, West Virginia & Fayetteville, North Carolina

- Counselor (1 year)
- Consulted with Nicky Cruz (of the movie and book *The Cross and The Switchblade* fame) on several occasions

Lost and Found Ministries
4th Avenue, Tucson, Arizona
—Founded by Ministers Pete and Mary Peterson

- Counselor (1 year)

CENTRUM of Hollywood
Hollywood, California

- Counselor with 24-hour help line
- Director of Hollywood Free Theater (that was to be opened on Hollywood Boulevard). Was selected over many applicants by the Board, which included Pat Boone, Catherine B. DeMill Quinn (Cecil B. DeMill's daughter and Anthony Quinn's wife), and Kleg Seth (Man-of-the-Year Award by Hollywood Chamber of Commerce and Director of CENTRUM), to name just three among other celebrities.

Youth with a Mission
Dallas (Walnut Hills/Bill Francis, Director) & Tyler, Texas

- Student trades craftsman
- Counselor
- Street ministry
- Consulted with Keith Green, Director of Last Days Ministries and musician
- Counseled with and received a life prophecy from Reverend David Wilkerson of Teen Challenge Programs. This handwritten prophecy is framed and hangs in my office:

    You have need of patience after you have done the will of the Father, that you might receive the promise.

    Be not denied. God is not mocked, whatsoever a man soweth, that he shall also reap. You have sown the seed you will reap in God's time.

    No weapon formed against you shall prosper. Greater is He that is within you than he that is within the world.

    If you do that which is right, who is he that can harm you?

    — Reverend David Wilkerson

Son Light Ministries
630 N. 4th Avenue, Tucson, Arizona

- Established first nonprofit organization and halfway house
- Ordained second time by Pastor Maynard Weisbrod of Calvary Evangelistic Center and Rev. David P. Strickland
- Spiritual Advisors
  - Rev. Tex Young, Jesus Fellowship
  - Rev. Ken Miles, Tucson Christian Fellowship
  - Rev. Gilbert Garcia, Son Life Church, Inc.
  - Rev. Gil Sandoval, Son Life Church, Inc.
- Worked with Pima County Jail pretrial release program under Director David Strickland, Department of Economic Security
- Volunteer Chaplain, Pima County Sheriff's Department for the County Jail (1977–1982), Reverend Dan Burgoyne, Head of Chaplain and affiliated with Grace Chapel Church

Global Community Communications Alliance and Divine Administration

Global Community Communications Alliance is a church supporting: a religious order and EcoVillage of 110+ international members living in community (with thousands of local and international supporters), Avalon Organic Gardens & EcoVillage, Personality Integration Rehabilitation Program for Teens and Adults, Global Family Legal Services, and many other ministries listed below. In addition Global Community Communications Alliance's supporting nonprofit organizations—Soulistic Medical Institute and Global Change Multi-Media—also support ministry programs listed below.

Founded in 1989 by Gabriel of Urantia (gabrielofurantia.info, gabrielofurantia.net, gabrielofurantia.com, gabrielofurantia.org) and Niánn Emerson Chase (niannemersonchase.org), Global Community Communications Alliance is located in southern Arizona in the charming, historic southwest towns of Tubac and Tumacácori—a sacred area known for centuries as "the Palm of God's Hand."

Find out more about our many local and global-related humanitarian efforts, services, and church programs:

Ministry Programs of Global Community Communications Alliance

Worldwide Sunday Services[SM]
Open to the public.
(520) 603-9932

Avalon Organic Gardens & EcoVillage[SM]
220-acre farm and ranch in southern Arizona,
using spiritually-based principles and
permaculture practices. Community Supported
Agriculture (CSA) provider.
avalongardens.org • (520) 603-9932

Personality Integration Rehabilitation Program[SM] **for Teens and Adults**
Assisting socially-disappointed souls
in their psychospiritual healing process.
pirp.info • (520) 603-9932

Friendly Hands Vocational Training[SM]
Spiritual Training Apprenticeship Programs in
a wide range of career fields.
(520) 603-9932

Global Family Legal Services[SM]
Legal aid in various fields focusing on immigration
for low-income individuals and families in need.
globalfamilylegalservices.org
(520) 398-3388 or (928) 282-2590

Homeless Is Not My Choice℠
Assisting the homeless or near homeless—(who are homeless because of an uncaring and insensitive government and corporate greed, foreclosures, and economic recession)—by providing housing, nutrition, hope, and vocation.
homelessisnotmychoice.org • (520) 603-9932

Spirit Steps℠ Tours
Offering enlightening tours for the seeking sojourner and eco-tourist.
spiritsteps.org
Toll-free (866) 508-0094
(520) 398-2655 or (928) 282-4562

Global Community Communications Schools of Ascension Science & The Physics of Rebellion℠
Teachings from the Continuing Fifth Epochal Revelation, *The URANTIA Book* and *The Cosmic Family* volumes.
gccschools.org • (520) 603-9932

Global Community Communications Schools for Teens and Children℠
The only school on the planet for teens and children incorporating the soul's point of universe origin and soul age, enabling the child to be guided into their correct destiny at a much younger age, bringing much earlier actualization, fulfillment, and self-confidence to the child.
gccschools.org • (520) 603-9932

Out of the Way Galleria℠

An eclectic blend of created art
contributed by local artisans and donors.
outofthewaygalleria.org • (520) 398-9409

Sacred Treasures℠

Clothing (men's & women's), arts & crafts
330 E. 7th Street, Tucson (4th Avenue area)
Sacred-Treasures.org • (520) 624-4418

Planetary Family Services℠

Provides services to create, embellish,
and bring Godly energy to your home environment.
planetaryfamilyservices.org
(520) 403-4207

Alternative Voice™

Periodical that addresses the many crises
of our world, fusing spirituality with activism.
alternativevoice.org • (520) 603-9932

Supporting Nonprofit Organizations

Soulistic Medical Institute℠ & Soulistic Hospice℠

Offers healthcare by professionals whose expertise
involves various healing modalities that encompass
the soul, mind, and body.
soulisticmedicalinstitute.org • (520) 398-3970

Soulistic Hospice • Tubac (520) 398-2333
soulistichospice.org • Tucson (520) 882-4111

Global Change Multi-Media℠
globalchangemultimedia.org
(520) 398-2542

Divisions of Global Change Multi-Media:

The Sea Of Glass — Center For The Arts℠
Venue – Music – Art – Dance – Multi Media – Theater – Healing Arts
Nonprofit organization
330 E. 7th Street, Tucson (4th Avenue area)
TheSeaOfGlass.org • (520) 490-2554

Future Studios℠
Recording studio.
futurestudios.org • (520) 398-2542

CosmoArt Studio℠
See artists' works-in-progress & art
330 E. 7th Street, Tucson (4th Avenue area)
CosmoArt.org • (520) 490-2554

Global Change Music℠
Nonprofit record label offers musicians recording opportunities using professional world-class equipment for voice and instrumental training.
globalchangemusic.org • (520) 398-2542

The Musicians That Need To Be Heard Network[SM]

Provides opportunities for musicians to communicate their music messages without spiritual compromise.
musiciansnet.org • (520) 398-2542

Global Change Television[SM]

Internet television station with a variety of programs of spiritual content, on demand.
globalchangetelevision.org
(520) 398-2542

Global Change Radio[SM]

Internet radio station offering on-demand audio webcasts, including talk radio on various religious and social themes.
globalchangeradio.org • (520) 398-2542

Music & Films at The Main Stage, Tubac and The Sea Of Glass,[SM] Tucson

Working with filmmakers and distributors of independent, activist, and educational films and documentaries that motivate spiritually thought-provoking group dialogue for the public. Booking national and international bands.
(520) 398-2542

Global Change Theater Company^{SM}
Dedicated to writing, performing, and staging plays
and various higher-consciousness, inspirational,
dramatic productions where students receive
training and opportunities to participate in
theatrical shows and workshops.
(520) 398-2542

**Global Change Multi-Media
Distribution Company**^{SM}
Distributes music, DVDs, books, magazines, and
any product that would be considered by its
parent company to be a Global Change Tool
for the dissemination of revelation and
spiritually-uplifting information
through media materials.

Global Change Multi-Media Productions^{SM}
Professional audio, video, and Internet service
producing spiritual and educational message media,
via Internet video streaming, live webcasting,
graphic design, and CD and video/DVD
media production.
(520) 398-2542

**Global Community
Communications Publishing**^{SM}
Publishing continuing epochal revelation
and related materials as well as
Global Change Teachings
and other spiritually-oriented texts.
gccpublishing.org • (520) 603-9932

Ministry Supporters

*Avalon Slow Food Enterprises
presents*

Food For Ascension[SM] Café
A farm-to-table restaurant
featuring plant-based foods, juices & teas.
330 E. 7th Street, Tucson (4th Avenue area)
FoodForAscension.org • (520) 882-4736

Global Community Communications Alliance

P.O. Box 4910, Tubac, AZ 85646 USA
(520) 603-9932

e-mail: info@gccalliance.org
gccalliance.org
globalchangetools.org

SEMINARS, WORKSHOPS & INTERNSHIPS

Earth Harmony Sustainability Seminars, Internships, & Workshops:

Green Building, Permaculture, Using Greenhouses To Extend The Growing Season, & Organic Gardening

- On survival in the near future, organic gardening, and the nuts and bolts of building an EcoVillage.

Held at Avalon Organic Gardens & EcoVillage in Tumacácori, Arizona
or
Held in your city

Contact (520) 603-9932
email: info@avalongardens.org
http://avalongardens.org

http://avalongardens.org/learn/seminars

Divine Administration Seminars
(for serious spiritual seekers)

- Weather Changes – Social – Political & Economic Disasters in Relationship to the Adjudication of the Bright & Morning Star versus Lucifer
- Protected and Safe Areas
- Could you be a Destiny Reservist?
- What is Epochal Revelation & the Importance of It?
  presented by Gabriel of Urantia and Niánn Emerson Chase
- Ascension Science and the Physics of Rebellion
  presented by Dr. Landau Lawrence, M.D.
- Starseed children in our midst: A case for multi-soul-age classrooms
  presented by Dr. Len'Mana Lee, Ed.D.
- Group encounter of the cosmic family
  presented by Dr. Marayeh Cunningham, Ph.D. Clinical Psychologist

Held at Avalon Organic Gardens & EcoVillage in Tumacácori, Arizona

Contact (520) 603-9932
email: info@gccalliance.org
http://gccalliance.org

http://gccalliance.org/divine-administration-seminars

ALLIANCE ORGANIZATIONS

The following organizations are allied in their efforts in some manner with the endeavors of Global Community Communications Alliance and Avalon Organic Gardens & EcoVillage.

ARANNOGALES (ASOCIACION DE REFORESTACION EN AMBOS NOGALES)

A joint effort of various organizations from both Nogales, Sonora and Nogales, Arizona who are dedicated to improving the quality of the air and the environment by re-establishing native vegetation.

BARRIO BREAD CO.

As a locally-grown business with a true passion for artisan bread making, Barrio Bread is a micro-bakery specializing in breads using ancient sourdough methods. Don Guerra (owner/baker) coached Avalon Gardens bakers using our earth oven. Our alliance with Don has been one of consultation and him drawing public attention to our sustainable food endeavors. Don was instrumental in assisting a film crew to visit Avalon Gardens to do a segment for a heritage grains documentary, specifically featuring Sonoran winter wheat we grow.

BORDER ACTION NETWORK

A human rights organization, based in Tucson, Arizona (about an hour north of the U.S./Mexico international border) whose mission is to establish safety, equality, dignity, understanding, and respect across cultures in border/immigrant communities. Executive Director Juanita Molina.

BORDER PATROL VICTIMS NETWORK

This Arizona-based activist group's intentions are to connect the families of people who have died during incidents with Border Patrol agents, calling for justice for families in the United States and Mexico. The organization is not focused solely on incidents in Southern Arizona, but across North America.

BORDERLANDS HABITAT RESTORATION INITIATIVE

A grassroots effort to maintain and enhance biodiversity in the Sky Island borderlands in Arizona/Sonora by first restoring physical processes, like stream flow, and then focusing on native plants and their pollinators that form the base of the "food chain" on which all other species depend. Avalon Organic Gardens hosts workshops and sets up educational demonstration sites with them.

BUENOS AIRES NATIONAL WILDLIFE REFUGE

Buenos Aires National Wildlife Refuge is 117,500-acre landscape that is part of the National Wildlife Refuge System in Altar Valley, focused on protecting and restoring habitat for wildlife. Prescribed burning, controlling exotic and invasive plants and animals, and erosion control are just some of the efforts taking place. Students from Global Community Communications Schools for Teens & Children have their environmental education booth at the Grasslands Fair at Buenos Aires annually in November.

COCHISE COMMUNITY COLLEGE

College students, as part of their "Sustainability Course," have come for several years for their education and credits for workshops with Avalon Organic Gardens & EcoVillage.

COMMUNITIES MAGAZINE

Global Community Communications Alliance (GCCA) has been listed in the Communities Directory since 1993. Articles from GCCA Co-Founder Niánn Emerson Chase and other members of the community have been published in Communities magazine. Some GCCA members have attended gatherings hosted by The Federation of Egalitarian Communities (the parent organization of Communities magazine).

COMMUNITY FOOD BANK OF SOUTHERN ARIZONA

Avalon Organic Gardens participates in events and farmers markets as community foods consignment program, as well as networking with them to improve community food security by promoting, demonstrating, advocating for, and collaboratively building an equitable and regional food system. The Community Food Bank supports farms, home gardening, farmers' markets, and youth programs that provide nutritional locally-grown foods and know-how to individuals and families interested in growing their own food. Avalon Gardens became certified and are able to accept FMNP (Farmers Market Nutrition Program) Vouchers and SFMNP (for seniors), WIC (Arizona Supplemental Nutrition Program for Women, Infants, and Children) Vouchers, SNAP (Supplemental Nutrition Assistance Program a.k.a. food stamps).

COSECHANDO BIENESTAR

Cosechando Bienestar (Harvesting Wellbeing) is a new initiative in Nogales, Arizona to promote the production, consumption, and awareness of local, healthy foods. The program promotes home and community gardens, the new Nogales Mercado, and other food enterprises. Community Garden Leaders receive in-depth instruction in gardening and food production led by Avalon Organic

Gardens. Community Garden Leaders work closely with staff at Mariposa Community Health Center (MCHC) to educate Nogales residents about vegetable gardening and food production.

EARTH DAY FESTIVAL

The Global Community Communications Schools for Teens & Children have participated in the Earth Day Festival at Reid Park in Tucson every year since 2009. We also have our Global Change Tools booth at the event annually.

FORGOTTEN POLLINATORS CAMPAIGN

Founded by Gary Nabhan, faculty member at the University of Arizona and an internationally-celebrated nature writer, food and farming activist, and proponent of conserving the links between biodiversity and cultural diversity. In 1995, the Arizona-Sonora Desert Museum, where Gary served as Director of Science, launched the Forgotten Pollinators Campaign, which helped focus international interest on threatened interactions between plants and their pollinators. Avalon Gardens works closely with Gary and is dedicated to educating people on the vital role pollinators play, offering workshops held at Avalon Organic Gardens & EcoVillage, including presenters such as Gary and Paul Kaiser.

FRIENDS OF THE SANTA CRUZ RIVER

Two community members of Global Community Communications Alliance (GCCA) sit on the Board of Friends of the Santa Cruz River (FOSCR), which is a highly respected Southern Arizona organization dedicated to preserving the flow, water quality, and banks of the Santa Cruz River. FOSCR does river advocacy through educational outreach programs as well as organizing river clean-ups of trash along the banks. Their River Watch program has been gathering and publishing scientific data on the Upper Basin of the Santa Cruz River since 1990 that is used by state & federal agencies to define the health of the river. GCCA has co-hosted events with FOSCR, including Celebrate the River, Junior Ranger Day (at Tumacácori National Historical Park) and the annual Celebrate the River Picnic and Youth Art Contest. Students from the Global Community Communications School's Bio-Regional Activism class participate in many FOSCR events, including presenting an educational outreach booth at events and assisting in the annual Fish Survey of the Santa Cruz River.

GLOBAL ECOVILLAGE NETWORK

Global Community Communications Alliance has been involved in the Community Sustainability Assessment process since 2001. Articles about the Avalon Organic Gardens & EcoVillage have been published on the

EcoVillage Network of the Americas newsletter, and people from this organization have visited Avalon Gardens.

GMO-FREE TUCSON

Provides education regarding the health risks of GMOs (Genetically Modified Organisms) in our food supply. Genetically modified organisms (GMOs) are plants or animals engineered to contain foreign DNA, usually from non-related species. They're in 80% of processed food in America. Global Community Communications Alliance works with activist and educator Jaime Hall and others at GMO-Free Tucson to help promote higher food choices, including through our all-organic GMO-free full-service restaurant: Food For Ascension Café in Tucson, Arizona.

INSTITUTO TECNOLOGICO DE NOGALES

In collaboration with Professor Diane Austin, Bureau of Applied Research in Anthropology, at the University of Arizona, civil engineers using recycled paper learn the theory and application of Papercrete, which provides affordable housing in Mexico.

MEXICAYOTL ACADEMY

Charter school in Nogales and Tucson that emphasizes Montessori philosophy, interculturlism, character leadership skills, and traditional dance. The children of Global Community Communications Schools For Teens & Children have interacted with their children and put on youth forums together. Avalon Organic Gardens & EcoVillage Master Gardeners and instructors taught students for several years how to garden, which led them to start their own school gardens.

NATIVE SEEDS/SEARCH

Conserves, distributes, and documents the adapted and diverse varieties of agricultural seeds, their wild relatives, and the role these seeds play in cultures of the American Southwest and northwest Mexico. Avalon Gardens has participated in several experiments and projects with Native Seeds/SEARCH.

NATURAL RESOURCES CONSERVATION SERVICE (NRCS)

Administers conservation programs in order to reduce soil erosion, enhance water supplies, improve water quality, increase wildlife habitat, and reduce damages caused by floods and other natural disasters. The Tucson office of the NRCS continues to collaborate closely with Avalon Organic Garden & EcoVillage staff on water conservation and air-quality programs.

NOGALES COMMUNITY DEVELOPMENT

Providing support for commercial revitalization and entrepreneurs, and affordable housing for families and individuals in Nogales, Arizona and Santa Cruz County.

PARAWATCHDOGS
(PATAGONIA AREA RESOURCE ALLIANCE)

The Patagonia Area Resource Alliance is a group that is working to protect the Patagonia Mountains from corporate mining. Members of Global Community Communications Alliance have attended their events and supported their efforts through networking and by publishing articles in local papers about the mining threats to the Patagonia Mountains.

PARTNERS FOR SUSTAINABLE POLLINATION

Partners for Sustainable Pollination (PFSP) works with farmers and beekeepers to improve the health of honey bees and support native pollinators. Avalon Organic Gardens has collaborated with Paul Kaiser—a Waldorf-inspired farmer and owner of Singing Frogs Farm in Sebastopol, California and winner of the 2010 Farmer-Rancher Award for the United States from the North American Pollinator Protection Campaign. Paul, along with Avalon Organic Gardens, are certified for gardeners of Bee Friendly Farming through PFSP.

RANCHO FELIZ

Rancho Feliz has worked on the border since 1987 and is a multi-national, secular, non-profit 501(c)(3) organization of volunteers committed to bucking the odds. However, Rancho Feliz is not welfare. Rather, they believe in the democratic redistribution of opportunity and the view that the best way to improve our own circumstances is to serve others. Thus they have changed thousands of lives on both sides of the border, with about 94% of every dollar raised going directly into their programs.

SABORES SIN FRONTERAS — FLAVORS WITHOUT BORDERS

A regional, bi-national and multi-cultural alliance to document, celebrate, and conserve farming and food folkways that span the U.S./Mexico borderlands from Texas and Tamaulipas on the east to Ambos Californias on the west.

SAHUARITA HIGH SCHOOL

Through a unique program, entitled Project Inspire, autistic students from Sahuarita High School (in Sahuarita, Arizona) spend time at Avalon Organic Gardens & EcoVillage working with the animals and gardening.

SANTA CRUZ COUNTY COMMUNITY FOUNDATION

The Santa Cruz Community Foundation (SCCF) identifies current and emerging border issues and mobilizes and strengthens community resources to solve these issues. The Foundation assists this unique border region to prepare for the future by strengthening, through grants and training, nonprofits (NPO) on both sides of the border. There is a diverse set of NPOs on the border ranging from job training programs, community centers, boys and girls clubs, arts groups, environmental restoration, agriculture, indigenous arts and culture, humane societies, libraries, children's homes, domestic violence abuse programs, migrant shelters, and soup kitchens that exist to alleviate the many inequalities and social and economic problems of the region.

SANTA CRUZ VALLEY CITIZENS COUNCIL

Santa Cruz Valley Citizens Council, Inc. (SCVCC) is a non-profit Arizona corporation whose purpose is to inform and educate its members about local and regional issues affecting the region. This is a group of citizens that really gets genuinely involved in local issues, and they have worked in the past to safeguard the region from overdevelopment and many other worthy causes. Some members of Global Community Communications Alliance belong to SCVCC and have been attending meetings and participating since 2008.

SAVE THE SCENIC SANTA RITAS

Save the Scenic Santa Ritas is a non-profit organization working to protect the Santa Rita and Patagonia Mountains from environmental degradation caused by mining and mineral exploration activities. Current activities are centered around the proposed Rosemont Copper Mine in the Santa Rita Mountains. Members of Global Community Communications Alliance have been supporting this organization since 2006 by tabling, participating in letter-writing campaigns, and engaging in the NEPA process to stop the Rosemont Copper Mine.

SIERRA CLUB — RINCON GROUP

The Tucson chapter of the Sierra Club, the Rincon Group, hosts many interesting events that members of Global Community Communications Alliance (GCCA) have attended. GCCA members also work with the Sierra Club in supporting certain campaigns that affect the regional physical and social environment.

SOMAS LA SEMILLA

"We Are The Seed" is a network of grassroots organizations, growers, clinics, and supporters in Arizona-Sonora borderlands creating alternative healthy food systems and sustainable agriculture practices. Avalon Gardens' Master Gardeners work in conjunction in many projects.

SONORAN INSTITUTE

Inspiring and enabling community decisions and public policies that respect the land and people of western North America; supporting resilient environmental and economic systems. Members of Global Community Communications Alliance (GCCA) work with the Sonoran Institute on the annual fish survey of the Santa Cruz River and other projects. The Sonoran Institute invited GCCA to contribute to the Santa Cruz County Water Harvesting Guidance Manual, which lists Water Harvesting Projects in Southeastern Arizona including the community's Avalon Gardens and Out-of-the-Way Galleria in Tubac. Members of the Sonoran Institute have participated in several tours of Avalon Gardens, as well as assisting with watershed management projects.

SOUTHWEST MARKETING NETWORK

The network's purpose is to help Southwestern producers and communities develop new and improved markets and enterprises and to rebuild local food systems.

TOHONO O'ODHAM NATION

We have an alliance with Bernard & Regina Siquieros of the Tohono O'Odham Nation. Bernard is the Educational Curator of the Tohono O'Odham Nation Cultural Center (in Sells, Arizona) and Regina is the Executive Assistant to the Chairman of the O'Odham Nation. They have come to Avalon Organic Gardens & EcoVillage to give presentations on their culture, and we have made reciprocal trips to visit them in Sells and Tucson.

T.R.E.A.T.Y. — TOTAL IMMERSION SCHOOL

Started by activist and actor Russell Means (one of the Co-Founders of A.I.M./American Indian Movement), the school is located at Porcupine, South Dakota on the Pine Ridge Sioux Reservation in Shannon Count—the poorest county in the United States. The concept of Culture Total Immersion Education has now spread worldwide. Indigenous peoples in Hawaii and Canada are creating their own Immersion Schools. The T.R.E.A.T.Y. Total Immersion School is the first for American Indians in the United States. Russell and Pearl Means have been good friends with Global Community Communications Alliance for many years. After Russell passed on in October 2012, his wife Pearl has continued her friendship with our community, including presenting "the

Russell Means Legacy" at The Sea of Glass in Spring 2014.

TUCSON MEET YOURSELF

A Tucson tradition, "folklife" festival with a focus on presenting artists and communities that carry on living traditions rooted in a group's own definition of identity, artistry, and cultural significance. Since 2007 Global Community Communications Alliance and Avalon Gardens have participated every year in this event, facilitating educational booths and workshops.

TUCSON PEACE FAIR AND CALENDAR

Avalon Gardens hosts an event on the Tucson Peace Calendar that is an invitation for people to come and work in the gardens during "Hands In The Soil" on the first Saturday morning of every month. This is followed by a discussion on Food Justice issues. Avalon Gardens also hosts an educational booth at the annual Peace Fair and provides some musicians for the entertainment venue.

TUCSON WATER FESTIVAL

The Global Community Communications Schools is a participant in the Tucson Water Festival. We share our educational displays on water with Friends of the Santa Cruz River and our Children's Choir has performed water songs at this unique event focused on water issues.

TUMACÁCORI NATIONAL HISTORICAL PARK

The mission ruins sites of San José de Tumacácori, Los Santos Ángeles de Guevavi, and San Cayetano de Calabazas are administered by Tumacácori National Historical Park. Avalon Organic Gardens & EcoVillage is right across the river from Tumacácori National Historical Park, and we have enjoyed many events with our neighbors at The Mission, including participating in the annual Fiesta and co-hosting Celebrate The River in 2009. Additionally our Spirit Steps Tours company accompanies guides and visitors to all tours of the Guevavi & San Cayetano mission sites.

UNIVERSITY OF ARIZONA

Faculty and students have been to Avalon Organic Gardens & EcoVillage for workshops to share and receive information, including with exchange students from South America.

WATERSHED MANAGEMENT GROUP

Watershed Management Group (WMG) develops community-based solutions to ensure the long-term prosperity of people and health of the environment, providing people with the knowledge, skills, and resources for sustainable livelihoods. Global Community Communications Alliance has enjoyed many activities with WMG, including assisting with the development of a watershed management project at Guy Tobin Trailhead in Rio Rico, Arizona, and many watershed management projects at Avalon Gardens in Tumacácori, Arizona.

WESTERN SARE (SUSTAINABLE AGRICULTURE RESEARCH AND EDUCATION)

A program of the U.S. Department of Agriculture that offers competitive grants conducted cooperatively by farmers, ranchers, researchers, and other agriculture professionals to advance farm and ranch systems that are profitable, environmentally sound, and good for communities. In collaboration with several grain growers we revived the production, milling, distribution, and marketing of the oldest extant grain variety adapted to the arid Southwest: White Sonora soft bread wheat.

WINDSONG PEACE & LEADERSHIP CENTER

An environmental education center fostering the connection between pressing environmental and social issues through state-of-the-art leadership and social issues training and focusing on reducing its impact on the environment. This year-round education center is committed to "leading by example," with advancements such as more than 70% of food grown on-site and sourced locally, rain-water harvesting, earthen building structures, and pollinator habitat restoration, as a grassroots role model for social and ecological regeneration. Windsong brings workshop participants to Avalon Gardens to tour and work, while teachers and students from Global Community Communications Schools for Teens & Children at Avalon Gardens attended a Social Justice Workshop at Windsong as well as a Me-To-We Activities Day.

WHY HUNGER?

Empowering 8,000+ community-based groups nationally, linking with international organizations advocating basic rights to food, land, water, & sustainable livelihoods. Founded in 1975 by the late musician Harry Chapin and Bill Ayres. Jen Chapin, Harry Chapin's daughter, has been to Avalon Gardens many times and presented workshops.

TO ORDER
globalchangetools.org
or TOLL-FREE **866-282-2205**

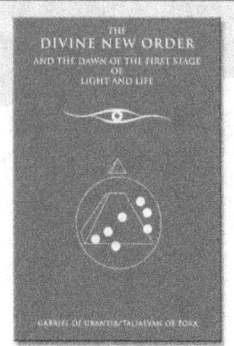

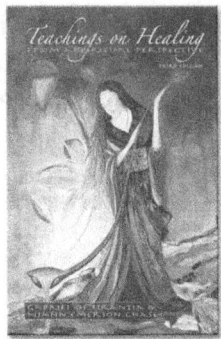

*Teachings on Healing
From a Spiritual Perspective*
135 pages
paperback $14.95
hardback $19.95

*The Divine New Order And
The Dawn Of The First
Stage Of Light And Life.*
400 pages
Gabriel of Urantia's
autobiography
BLACK & WHITE PHOTOS
paperback $14.95
hardback $21.95
COLOR PHOTOS
paperback $22.95
hardback $30.95

The Cosmic Family, Volumes I and II
Ascension Science & The Physics of Rebellion

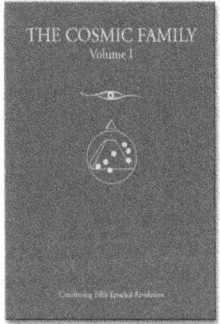

The Continuation of
The URANTIA Book

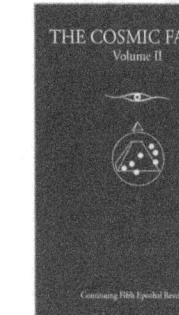

Volume I - 393 pages
paperback $29.95
hardback $39.95

Volume II - 567 pages
paperback $34.95
hardback $49.95

TO ORDER
globalchangetools.org
or TOLL-FREE 866-282-2205

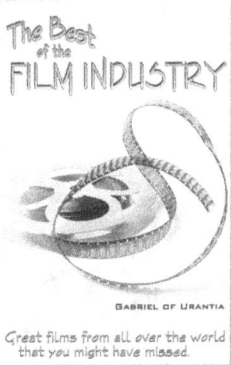

Great films from all over the world that you might have missed.

The industry only promotes what it feels is "box office", and box office is usually sensationalized trash.

More than 1,254 film reviews
paperback $13.95

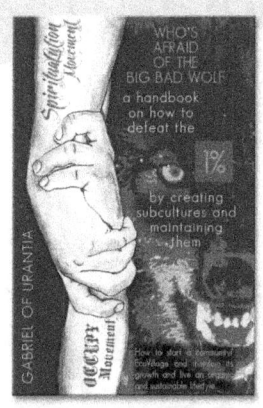

Who's Afraid Of The Big Bad Wolf?
—A Handbook On How To Defeat The 1% By Creating Subcultures And Maintaining Them
240 pages

paperback $14.95
hardback $19.95

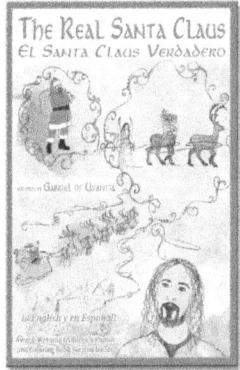

Your children will love the connect between Jesus and Santa (in English y en Español)
hardback $19.95

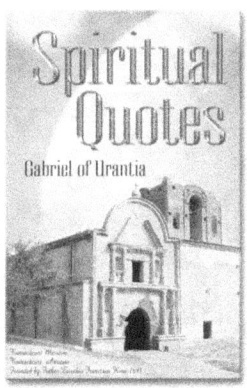

Quotes that will enrich your life
paperback $8.95

TO ORDER
globalchangetools.org
or Toll-Free **866-282-2205**

CosmoPop® Music
Lyrical and Melodic Masterpieces

TALIASVAN
& The Bright & Morning Star Band

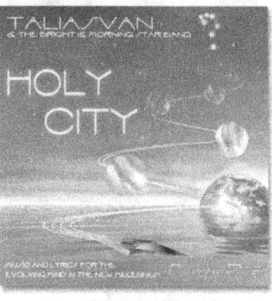

Holy City
CosmoRock, CosmoFolk,
& CosmoCountry
65 min $17.95

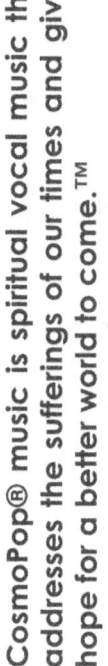

CosmoPop® music is spiritual vocal music that addresses the sufferings of our times and gives hope for a better world to come.™

CosmoPop Millennium
65 min $17.95

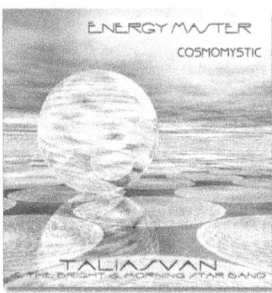

Energy Master CosmoMystic
$21.95 CD and DVD set
$16.95 CD only
CD 58 min / DVD 60 min

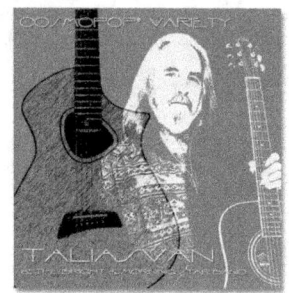

CosmoPop Variety
CosmoRock, CosmoFolk,
CosmoMystic, & CosmoCountry
76 min $18.95

Gabriel of Urantia is also known as TaliasVan
& The Bright & Morning Star Band with his music career.

TO ORDER
globalchangetools.org
or Toll-Free 866-282-2205

TALIASVAN
& The Bright & Morning Star Band

CosmoPop® Music
Lyrical and Melodic Masterpieces

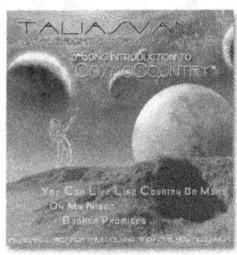

3-song introduction to
CosmoCountry
19 min $10.95

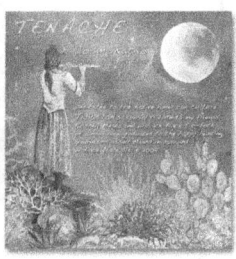

Tenache 3-song
CosmoNative
32 min $11.95

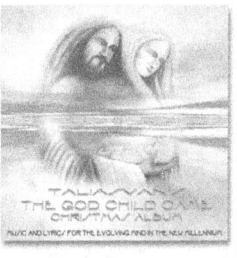

The God Child Came
Christmas CD
75 min $18.95

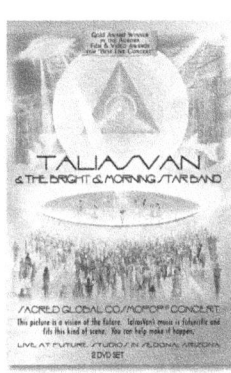

Sacred Global CosmoPop
Concert DVD 2-disc set
Live at Future Studios
in Sedona
2 hr 15 min $22.95

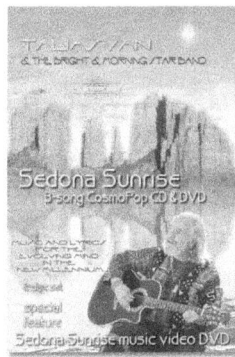

Sedona Sunrise
3 song CosmoPop
CD / DVD set
CD 17 min / DVD 7 min
$11.95

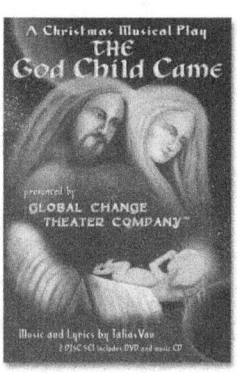

The God Child Came
Christmas Play & CD
CD / DVD set
CD 75 min / DVD 75 min
$22.95

TO ORDER
globalchangetools.org
or TOLL-FREE **866-282-2205**

TALIASVAN'S
45-VOICE BRIGHT & MORNING STAR CHOIR & ORCHESTRA

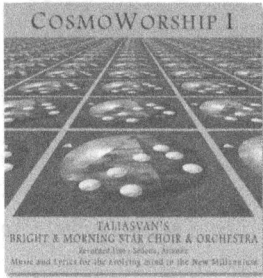

CosmoWorship I
58 min $13.95

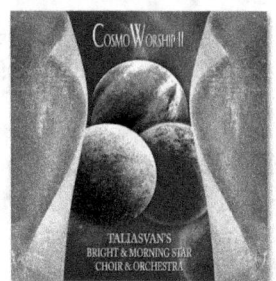

CosmoWorship II
72 min $14.95

other GLOBAL CHANGE MUSIC bands

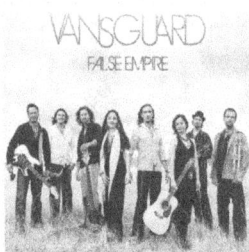

VansGuard
False Empire
46 min $15.95

Starseed Acoustic Ensemble
Interuniversal Home
60 min $12.95

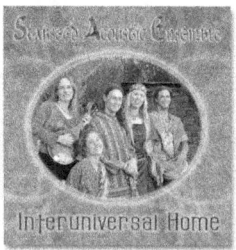

Other titles by Gabriel of Urantia
available from
Global Community Communications Publishing
A Division of Global Change Multi-Media

*The Divine New Order And
The Dawn Of The First Stage Of Light And Life*
by Gabriel of Urantia
Autobiography of Gabriel of Urantia and
the history of the beginning of
Global Community Communications Alliance.

The Cosmic Family, Volume I
as transmitted through Gabriel of Urantia
Continuing Fifth Epochal Revelation,
Papers 197–228 succeeding *The URANTIA Book.*

The Cosmic Family, Volume II
as transmitted through Gabriel of Urantia
Continuing Fifth Epochal Revelation, Papers 229–261
succeeding *The Cosmic Family, Volume I.*

Messages To Urantia, 1997–2000
as transmitted through Gabriel of Urantia
A collection of 19 sacred messages from celestial beings
addressing the state of our world, Urantia.

Teachings On Healing, From A Spiritual Perspective
by Gabriel of Urantia and Niánn Emerson Chase
Teachings focused on bringing about healing
on the physical, mental, emotional, and spiritual levels.

*The Best Of The Film Industry
—Movies You Don't Want To Miss!*
compiled by Gabriel of Urantia
A detailed list of commentaries and reviews of films
that educate, challenge, and expand the consciousness.

***Making The Most Of Media Exposure For Global Change
Versus Our Experience With The Media***
by Gabriel of Urantia and Niánn Emerson Chase
Firsthand account of experiences with
corporate-controlled media.

Spiritual Quotes
by Gabriel of Urantia
A collection of spiritual insights and wisdom
addressing many of life's facets.

The Real Santa Claus
by Gabriel of Urantia
A children's book sharing a unique perspective on
who really is the beloved Santa/St. Nicholas of Christmas.

***Who's Afraid Of The Big Bad Wolf?
— A Handbook On How To Defeat The 1%
By Creating Subcultures and Maintaining Them***
by Gabriel of Urantia
A collection of articles addressing deeper issues in
the Occupy / 99% movement with viable solutions.
Includes a wonderful photo gallery
of Global Change Multi-Media attending
Occupy events around the country.

Upcoming Books (Works In Progress)

The Cosmic Family, Volumes III, IV and *V*

*Spiritual Qualities, Virtues, And Non-Virtues,
And Other Spiritual Critiques*

*Guide To Healing Various Ailments, Based On Symptoms
Of Urantians (New Souls) And Starseed (Older Souls)*

The Fall From The Bright Star

*The Food For Ascension™ Cookbook
For Urantians And Starseed*